Qualitative Research for Allied Health Professionals: Challenging Choices

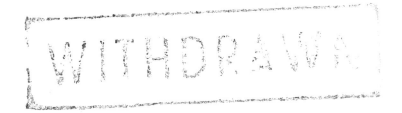

D1428754

Qualitative Research for Allied Health Professionals: Challenging Choices

Edited by

Linda Finlay and Claire Ballinger

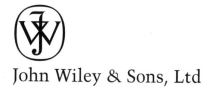

John Wiley & Sons, Ltd

Email (for orders and customer service enquiries): cs-books@wiley.co.uk
Visit our Home Page on www.wiley.com

Other Wiley Editorial Offices

John Wiley & Sons Inc., 111 River Street, Hoboken, NJ 07030, USA

Jossey-Bass, 989 Market Street, San Francisco, CA 94103-1741, USA

Wiley-VCH Verlag GmbH, Boschstr. 12, D-69469 Weinheim, Germany

John Wiley & Sons Australia Ltd, 42 McDougall Street, Milton, Queensland 4064, Australia

John Wiley & Sons (Asia) Pte Ltd, 2 Clementi Loop #02-01, Jin Xing Distripark, Singapore 129809

John Wiley & Sons Canada Ltd, 22 Worcester Road, Etobicoke, Ontario, Canada M9W 1L1

Wiley also publishes its books in a variety of electronic formats. Some content that appears in print may not be available in electronic books.

Library of Congress Cataloging-in-Publication Data
Qualitative research for allied health professionals : challenging choices / edited by Linda Finlay and Claire Ballinger.
     p.   ;   cm.
     Includes bibliographical references and index.
     ISBN-13: 978-0-470-01963-4 (pbk. : alk. paper)
     ISBN-10: 0-470-01963-8 (pbk. : alk. paper)
     1. Qualitative research.   2. Medicine – Research – Methodology.   3. Medical care – Research – Methodology.   4. Allied health personnel.
     [DNLM: 1. Allied Health Occupations.   2. Qualitative Research.
W 21.5 Q15 2006]   I. Finlay, Linda, 1957–   II. Ballinger, Claire.
     R853.Q34Q83 2006
     610'.72 – dc22
                                                                                            2005025318

A catalogue record for this book is available from the British Library
ISBN-13   978-0-470-01963-4
ISBN-10   0-470-01963-8
Printed and bound in Great Britain by TJ International Ltd, Padstow, Cornwall

This book is printed on acid-free paper responsibly manufactured from sustainable forestry in which at least two trees are planted for each one used for paper production.

For Abbi, Amy and Anthony

Contents

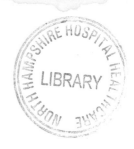

Contributors

Linda Finlay PhD, BA(Hons), DipCOT, Academic Consultant, The Open University, Milton Keynes and MSc dissertation supervisor Physiotherapy & OT, University of East London, UK.

Claire Ballinger PhD, MSc, DipCOT, Reader in Occupational Therapy, London South Bank University, UK.

Tanya Campbell-Breen PhD, MSc, BSc (OT), Lecturer, Queen Margaret University College, Edinburgh, UK.

Julianne Cheek PhD, Professor and Director, Early Career Researcher Development, School of Health Sciences, University of South Australia, Australia.

Michael Curtin, EdD, MPhil, BOccThy, Course Coordinator and Senior Lecturer, Occupational Therapy, School of Community Health, Charles Sturt University, NSW, Australia.

Sarah G. Dean PhD, MSc, BSc(Hons), DipCSP, Senior Lecturer in Rehabilitation, Department of Medicine, Wellington School of Medicine and Health Sciences, University of Otago, Wellington, New Zealand.

Paula Hyde PhD, MBA, BSc(Hons), Lecturer in leadership and experiential learning, Manchester Business School, University of Manchester, UK.

Anne Killett, MA, DipCOT, School of Allied Health Professions, University of East Anglia, UK.

Ruth H. Parry PhD, MMedSci, MCSP, Postdoctoral Research Fellow and Research Physiotherapist, Institute of Work, Health and Organisations, University of Nottingham, UK.

Sheila Payne PhD, CPsychol, BA(Hons), RN, DipN Professor in Palliative Care, Palliative and End-of-Life Care Research Group, University of Sheffield, UK.

Fiona Poland PhD, MA Econ, BA Econ (Hons), Senior Lecturer in Therapy Research, School of Allied Health Professions, University of East Anglia, UK.

Barbara Richardson PhD, MSc, FCSP, Reader, Physiotherapy, School of Allied Health Professions, Institute of Health, University of East Anglia, Norwich, UK.

Jonathan A. Smith DPhil, MSc, BA Reader in Psychology, Birkbeck, University of London, UK.

Mandy Stanley MHSc(OT), BAppSc(OT), Lecturer, Occupational Therapy programme, School of Health Sciences, University of South Australia, Adelaide, Australia.

Barbara Steward PhD, MA, BA, TDipCOT, Cert Ed(FE), Senior Lecturer/Course Leader, Lincolnshire Work Based Learning Programme in Occupational Therapy, Sheffield Hallam University, UK.

Rose Wiles PhD, BSc, Principal Research Fellow, ESRC National Centre for Research Methods, University of Southampton, UK.

Prologue

SUPERVISOR: So how are your ideas for your research coming along?

STUDENT: I thought I might like my study to focus on exploring pain.

SUPERVISOR: OK. Do you mean you want to hear about individuals' experience of pain? Or how people perceive and represent their pain? Or maybe you want to focus on how pain is constructed? Your research question is really important as it implies different methodologies.

STUDENT: Oh, definitely the first. The people I work with in therapy have such vivid ways of talking about their pain. I don't think we really appreciate what it's like.

SUPERVISOR: That's interesting. You could do that. But think for a minute. There are a number of assumptions you seem to be making here: that people's experience of pain is a real entity; that they have a way of describing it; and that you will be able to capture what that is.

STUDENT: Umm, yes, I guess so. (*Hesitation*) I'm not sure I really understand what you're saying.

SUPERVISOR: You seem to be suggesting that pain is an experience that's clear-cut and absolute. Many qualitative researchers would see the experience of pain not as cut and dried but as highly variable. They'd argue that what we really need to investigate is people's *meanings* of pain: what pain means to individuals will vary according to the context and their needs at the time. So you might want to think about that. Patients will be presenting themselves to you in a certain light. Where you talk to them, and in what capacity, might make a difference to what they say.

STUDENT: Well, I hadn't thought of that. (*Pause*) I suppose that means they might say something different, for example if a family member rather than a therapist were to ask them about it?

SUPERVISOR: Absolutely. Your challenge is to decide what exactly you think you mean by 'experience of pain', and then you need to think about how best to explore it. So far, you've only alluded to interviews as a possible method of data collection, or data generation as I prefer to call it. Let's play around with some other possible ways of generating data. Can you think of any?

STUDENT: Hmm. That's difficult. I suppose I had assumed that talking to people would be the most obvious way of getting at what it was like for them.

SUPERVISOR: Well, I'm not suggesting that you don't do interviews. At this stage, all I'm asking is that you keep open to different possibilities. How about asking people to write diaries, for example . . .

Does this conversation sound familiar? The idea of writing this book sprang in part from our past participation in such discussions. Initially, we took part as students who were about to embark on specific qualitative research journeys. Latterly, we have participated as teachers and supervisors, guiding others through the dense tangle of qualitative approaches, paradigms and methodologies. Whether as apprehensive student or experienced teacher, however, we share an enthusiasm and a passion for qualitative modes of enquiry: a commitment that we hope, in the pages of this book, to convey to our readers.

This book is also a celebration of the 'coming of age' of the allied health professions (AHPs) within the qualitative research arena. AHP researchers are now able to engage in debate on methodology and epistemology in a way that would have been impossible even ten years ago. This is evidenced by the large number of therapists embarking on higher degrees, the contribution of therapy researchers to international generic research publications such as the journal *Qualitative Health Research*, and extensive thoughtful discussion within our professional journals.

Quite deliberately, the subtitle of this book, *Challenging Choices*, carries a double meaning. It makes the point that the qualitative research endeavour is likely to be challenging to us as researchers. But it also affirms that the choices that we make in designing, carrying out and reporting our research will be challenged and contested. These are themes we focus on in this book. Specifically, our aims are to:

- highlight some of the choices that you as the researcher will be required to make, and clarify their implications;

- offer a wide range of practical examples to show how these different ways of doing qualitative research can be managed;
- critically examine a variety of qualitative research methodologies of particular interest to allied health professionals;
- make explicit the links between epistemology, methodology and method.

This book is structured in three parts. In Part I, we aim to sensitise you, the reader, to the complex issues that challenge qualitative researchers at the planning stage of their projects. In Part II, the challenge of using different methodologies in practice is critically explored by 15 authors who share their individual research experiences. Part III examines the choices we make when we evaluate and present research.

We hope you will find this book both exciting and helpful. Inevitably, there are many gaps in terms of topics and issues covered, and methodologies represented. Although we want the book to have a practical focus, we do not offer detailed guidelines about specific methods. Instead, we provide examples from a broad sweep of research practice in an attempt to promote critical dialogue.

As our contributing authors reveal their struggles and uncertainties, we value their preparedness to be open. We continue to be impressed by their thoughtfulness, their concern for participants and ethical practice, and their commitment to qualitative research. We also celebrate the diversity demonstrated across these contributions as the authors reveal different values, theoretical perspectives and methodological commitments.

Many people have helped with the successive drafts of this book. First, we'd like to acknowledge the rich contribution made by Barbara Steward, who played a key role in conceiving this project. Secondly, we are indebted to all our chapter authors. They rose to the challenge of writing about their research within tight word limits and showed patience and grace in the face of our shifting ideas for chapter structure. Thirdly, we'd like to acknowledge our husbands Mel and Chris: without their support and encouragement we couldn't have carried the project through. Then, a special thanks goes to Susan Ram for her invaluable editing advice. Finally, our gratitude needs to be extended to Colin Whurr for initially believing in the project and to Emma Hatfield (Project Editor) and her team for seeing the manuscript through to publication.

Linda Finlay and Claire Ballinger
September 2005

PART I

Planning the Research

In this first part of the book, we invite you to reflect on issues and questions that arise during the planning phase of research. The first of these is whether an exploratory, qualitative approach to your topic of interest is the best way forward. In **Chapter 1**, Linda Finlay takes a look at the diverse methodologies that are included within the broad church of qualitative research. She also clarifies the sorts of questions that qualitative research approaches are particularly suited to answering.

Novice researchers are often bewildered by the plethora of terms and expressions they encounter in their preliminary reading around qualitative research approaches. In **Chapter 2**, Linda Finlay sets out to demystify concepts such as 'methodology', 'epistemology' and 'ontology'. Using examples from practice, she shows how methodology and method are inter-related, and illustrates how initial choices have consequences for the interpretation of data and for the types of explanation adopted.

Chapter 3, by Barbara Steward, continues to explore the decisions related to research method with which a qualitative researcher must engage. She offers practical advice on a range of questions, including how to choose a research topic and question, how to use supporting literature, which methods to choose, and how to find and gain access to participants.

The parameters of what is considered principled research have undergone change, with important consequences for research. In **Chapter 4**, the final one in this opening part of the book, Claire Ballinger and Rose Wiles look at some of the issues relating to research ethics and governance. They offer suggestions for how to interpret current guidelines to suit qualitative enquiry.

1

'Going Exploring': The Nature of Qualitative Research

LINDA FINLAY

The process of engaging in qualitative research is rather like 'going exploring'. Uncharted territory beyond the reach of conventional research (with its claims to objectivity and its quantitative instincts) beckons us irresistibly. We embark on a 'quest' (Rosaldo, 1989); we sense that 'adventure' (Willig, 2001) lies ahead. Our preparations made, we begin our research journey with no fixed ideas about its content or destination. If anything, we expect to be surprised; we know that, for all our planning, we will stumble into unanticipated situations or tread unmapped paths. What we discover along the way may astonish, delight or perplex us. We may lose our way, go round in circles, find solid ground giving way to mire, it matters not. The qualitative research journey remains enticing though 'full of muddy ambiguity and mul- tiple trails as researchers negotiate the swamp of interminable decon- structions, self analysis and self disclosure' (Finlay, 2002, p. 209).

Like explorers bent on penetrating the unknown, qualitative researchers are fired by the excitement and challenge of the enterprise. Frustration and discomfort are more than counterbalanced by mo- ments of exhilaration. The challenge lies in mapping a path, with the help of compass and guides (books, mentors and supervisors), that safe- guards our passage while enabling us to experience the richness and complexity of our research terrain.

The chapters in this book aim to reveal something of the excitement and satisfactions of *doing* qualitative research, along with the uncer-

Qualitative Research for Allied Health Professionals: Challenging Choices. Edited by Linda Finlay and Claire Ballinger.   Copyright 2006 by John Wiley & Sons Ltd.   ISBN 0-470-01963-8.

....nties and frustrations. More specifically, the authors who come together in this volume seek to highlight some of the 'challenging choices' they have had to face. There are many routes through – many ways of doing – qualitative research, and this very diversity means that decisions need to be carefully thought through. The purpose of this book is to contribute to making well-considered choices.

CHALLENGING CHOICES

One early critical choice that qualitative researchers face when planning research is which of the great variety of qualitative **methodologies** to adopt. As Cresswell (1998, p. 4) observes, qualitative researchers have before them 'a baffling number of choices of traditions'! Should the research be conducted on the basis of grounded theory? Or should the choice be ethnomethodology? Or discourse analysis? Or phenomenology? Or ethnography? These are just a few of the diverse options. More than just selecting a methodology, we need to think about the aim and focus of our research. If we want to explore individuals' life experiences, then our options would orientate towards phenomenological, psychodynamic, biographical or narrative research (such as described in Chapters 9, 10, 11 and 12). If the focus is to be more on talk or text, then discourse or conversation analysis would be the better choice (see Chapters 8 and 14). If the aim is to understand cultural practices, then we would opt for ethnography (Chapter 6) or case-study research on organisations (Chapter 15).

The next set of decisions relates to the **methods** we will use to collect, and then analyse, data. What sources of data are potentially available and appropriate? Which methods of data collection and analysis would be most suitable, given our chosen methodology? Should we opt for interviews, observation or other procedures to gather data? Would combining methods (see Chapter 7) offer something more? What can the chosen methods feasibly tell us? Should our analysis take the form of a descriptive narrative (see Chapter 13) or should it be organised thematically (for instance in the grounded theory discussed in Chapter 5)? Given the inevitable constraints of time and competing demands, what is the most practical option?

In focusing on methodology and method, questions are raised about our **epistemological** and **theoretical** stance (see Chapter 2). For example, we should be in no confusion as to whether we are taking a realist or relativist position or whether we are attempting to describe or explain the social world. Reaching a clear stance in relation to such questions is by no means easy. As two experienced researchers have noted, qualitative research 'embraces within its own multiple disciplinary histories constant tensions and contradictions over the project itself, including its methods and the forms its findings and interpretations take' (Denzin and Lincoln, 1994, p. 4).

There are also decisions to be made about **ethics** and the kinds of **relationships** we want to develop with our participants (see Chapters 3 and 4) and/or the readers and consumers of our research. Given that there is an 'intimate relationship between the researcher and what is studied' (Denzin and Lincoln, 1994, p. 4), what is our role as researcher? Beyond seeking to do no harm, we often aim to empower and 'give voice' to our participants. We must be mindful that our research – which encourages us to reflect on ourselves and the social world around us – has the potential to be transformative, changing both us and our participants. If such power exists within our research, then that needs to be managed and respected. A key question here is whose interests are served by our research?

Finally, we need to think about how we should **evaluate** and **present** our research (see Chapters 16 and 17). How can this be done to ensure that our work is responsible and has integrity, meaning and value? As Seale points out:

> A fallibilistic approach ... is not well served by presenting a personal interpretation and then simply saying that people are free to disagree if they so wish. It requires a much more active and labour-intensive approach towards genuinely self-critical research, so that something of originality and value is created. (Seale, 1999, p. 6)

The choices we make inevitably lead us along different paths into varied explorations of contrasting terrains. Our versions of qualitative research will vary considerably. For all that, however, there are similarities to be found in the territory we explore and the navigational tools we use to guide us and give us direction. There are basic tenets or commonalities that unite seemingly disparate qualitative methodologies.

COMMONALITIES

If you put all the authors of this book in the same room it would probably be a noisy affair! We would fiercely debate the nature of the social world (ontology) and we'd argue about the best way to study it. Not all of us would agree on the objective existence of a social world for us to study in the first place. Some would argue that it is the meanings, interpretations and language we use that construct that world. Some qualitative researchers would aim for objective, systematic research that reflects the social world as much as possible. Others disagree, valuing instead the existence of multiple realities and subjectivities and the potential of the research to transform what is being studied. In these ways, we would bandy words and concepts, contesting their meanings. (A quick look at the glossary at the end of the book will give you an indication of the sorts of ambiguities we face here.)

For all our passionate (but friendly) disagreement, however, we respect one another's choices. And we're also conscious of sharing certain assumptions, which distinguish us in a fundamental way from researchers in the quantitative, positivist tradition. To a greater or lesser extent, qualitative researchers all acknowledge and value

- the central role played by the researcher in the construction of knowledge;
- the significance of the researcher's relationship with participants and/or the social world;
- inductive, exploratory, hypothesis-generating rather than hypothesis-testing research;
- the role of interpretation and emergent meanings;
- the complex, rich and messy nature of qualitative findings.

These ideas are briefly explored below.

THE RESEARCHER'S ROLE IN THE CONSTRUCTION OF KNOWLEDGE

Qualitative researchers accept that the researcher is a central figure who influences, and perhaps actively constructs, the collection, selection and interpretation of data. Researcher subjectivity – called 'bias' in quantitative research – is celebrated rather than seen as something to be shunned; it is viewed as an opportunity rather than a problem (Finlay, 2002).

THE SIGNIFICANCE OF THE RESEARCHER'S RELATIONSHIPS

We recognise that research is co-constituted, a joint product of participants, researchers and readers, and the relationship they build. Our participants affect us, just as we affect them. We also recognise that we are influenced by wider social relationships and our historical and cultural situatedness in the world – and this recognition is subsumed into our work.

THE INDUCTIVE, EXPLORATORY, HYPOTHESIS-GENERATING NATURE OF QUALITATIVE RESEARCH

Qualitative researchers start with open research questions rather than having a hypothesis to test. Qualitative research aims to investigate and understand the social world rather than to predict, explain and control behaviour. The focus is on the 'how' and 'what' rather than 'why' and 'whether'. For instance, instead of investigating whether a treatment intervention is effective by comparing a treatment group with a control group, the qualitative researcher would ask: 'How does this client experience this treatment?'

THE ROLE OF MEANINGS AND INTERPRETATION

We are concerned with how people make sense of the world and how they experience events. 'Qualitative researchers study things in their natural settings, attempting to make sense of or interpret phenomena in terms of the meanings people bring to them' (Denzin and Lincoln, 1994, p. 2). We understand that meanings are fluid, subject to interpretation, and are negotiated within particular social contexts. We acknowledge that other researchers, using the same data, are likely to unfold different stories.

THE COMPLEX, RICH AND MESSY NATURE OF QUALITATIVE FINDINGS

Qualitative researchers believe in rich, textured description that has the potential to move others. At the same time we recognise that findings are always partial, tentative, ambiguous, fluid and open to multiple interpretations and emergent meanings. We see our social world as too chaotic to be represented in unambiguous, clear-cut ways, or in terms of cause and effect. Whatever methodology qualitative researchers choose to embrace, we embark on a journey that is endlessly fascinating: a potentially transformative exploration of relationships and meanings within our social world. Whatever we know of our world, the qualitative research journey opens fresh horizons, showing us how much more lies waiting to be explored.

REFERENCES

Cresswell, J.W. (1998) *Qualitative Inquiry and Research Design: Choosing Among Five Traditions*, Thousand Oaks: Sage Publications.

Denzin, N.K. and Lincoln, Y.S. (eds) (1994) *Handbook of Qualitative Research*, Thousand Oaks: Sage Publications.

Finlay, L. (2002) 'Negotiating the swamp: The opportunity and challenge of reflexivity in research practice', *Qualitative Research*, 2(2): 209–30.

Rosaldo, R. (1989) *Culture and Truth: Renewing the Anthropologist's Search for Meaning*, Boston: Beacon.

Seale, C. (1999) *The Quality of Qualitative Research*, London: Sage Publications.

Willig, C. (2001) *Introducing Qualitative Research in Psychology: Adventures in Theory and Method*, Buckingham: Open University Press.

2

Mapping Methodology

LINDA FINLAY

Novice researchers planning their research projects can all too easily make the mistake of adopting a specific method (for instance doing interviews) without first locating that method in terms of a broader methodology, namely philosophy and associated methods. This is like embarking on a qualitative research 'adventure' (to pick up the theme in Chapter 1) without planning, preparation or a map!

This chapter seeks to provide a 'map' of the methodological choices facing researchers who embark on qualitative research. Specifically, I explore how methodology is always underpinned by philosophical and theoretical ideas (be they implicit or explicit) and how data collection and analysis methods tend to flow naturally from these methodologies. If we are truly to get to grips with qualitative research, it is crucial to be clear about the ideas we're embracing when we commit to a methodology.

The idea of a chapter on philosophy and theory could well turn some readers off. If this is your reaction, I'd ask you to bear with me. I want to share my enthusiasm and commitment to this way of thinking about methodology. I hope to show you how meaningful and important philosophy and theory are – at the very least, that it is essential to be aware of possible options. Qualitative researchers need to be able to understand such concepts as epistemology, interpretivism, relativism and reflexivity. These are concepts that we regularly confront when reading qualitative research papers and when discussing our work with others. Grappling with these meanings transforms our research.

Qualitative Research for Allied Health Professionals: Challenging Choices. Edited by Linda Finlay and Claire Ballinger.   Copyright 2006 by John Wiley & Sons Ltd.   ISBN 0-470-01963-8.

The first section of the chapter describes some different methodologies and explores the links between methodology and method. Then the next two sections, on philosophy and theory respectively, demonstrate how all research is underpinned by ideas, beliefs and assumptions. Finally, a reflections section emphasises that in a context of messy practice and contested ideas, it becomes even more important to attend to the goals and peculiarities of your specific methodology.

CHOOSING YOUR METHODOLOGY

COMMITTING TO A METHODOLOGY

Methodology is the overarching approach to research and encompasses both philosophy and methods (see Figure 2.1). Choosing a methodol-

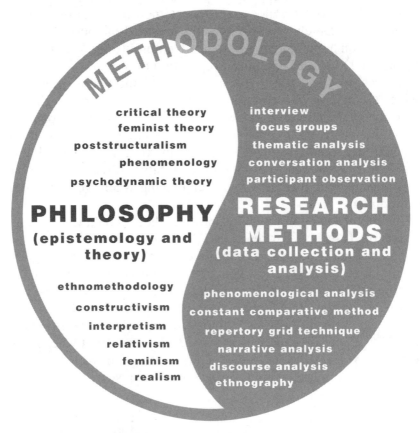

Figure 2.1 Methodology bridging philosophy and method

ogy means selecting from alternative philosophical or theoretical positions, and deciding what research methods (procedures to collect and analyse data) to use. Philosophy and research methods are intertwined. Choosing particular philosophies usually implies the use of particular methods and vice versa.

There are abundant methodological approaches on offer: ethnomethodology, ethnography, phenomenology, grounded theory, discourse analysis, narrative analysis, feminist approaches, cooperative enquiry, case studies, repertory grid, action research, biographical and historical approaches, and so on. (See the glossary for an orientating description of some of these key methodologies.) Each of these methodologies carries different aims, involves different research designs and utilises different research methods.

The examples in Box 2.1 demonstrate how five researchers aim to conduct and analyse their research in different ways – ways that

---

Box 2.1   Research on living with disability: five methodologies

Five researchers all plan to interview six participants on how they live and cope with their disability.

Niall chooses to do a **grounded theory** study underpinned by 'postpositivist', realist assumptions. His interview questions are focused analytically on the 'coping' process. When and how does coping happen? What disrupts coping? He sees the participants' responses as a reasonably accurate reflection of their thoughts and feelings. He aims to categorise systematically their types of coping and to show how coping occurs in particular social situations. As he analyses the emergent themes, he works hard to stay faithful to what is contained in the data and not let personal biases intrude.

Julie adopts a **phenomenological** approach, aiming for rich description of individuals' lived experience. She asks her participants to describe a particular moment of living with their disability as concretely as possible and she then focuses on what it means to them personally. She analyses this data hermeneutically in terms of existential themes, exploring her participants' sense of embodiment, self–other relations, time and space. Her study is underpinned by 'critical realist' assumptions: she assumes that the participants' accounts reflect something of their subjective perceptions of their lived experience while also recognising that her own interpretations have, inevitably, played a crucial role.

Masha undertakes a **discourse analysis**, based on social constructionist ideas. She aims to examine the way 'disability' is both constructed and performed by individuals. She views the 'text' (her transcripts) as a manifestation of discursive resources on which the participants are drawing to construct their versions. She is alert to the presence of cultural scripts, such as the use of particular narratives and metaphors (for example, seeing disability as 'personal tragedy' or 'heroic quest'). She takes her reflexive analysis seriously by recognising the power of her role as interviewer and the entirely co-constructed nature of the text. By acknowledging that another researcher would have obtained a different 'story', she demonstrates her 'relativist' assumptions.

Johnson undertakes an **ethnographic** study, aiming to understand the culture and characteristics of a rehabilitation unit as a social setting geared to helping clients with their disabilities. His interview questions are focused on how the clients perceive themselves and their rehabilitation. He is interested in how the clients are positioned in the setting and how they interact with each other and the professionals. He aims to develop a story of these clients and how this particular social and cultural context enables clients to live positively with their disability. By recognising the multiplicity of voices within a specific culture, he is taking an explicitly 'relativist' stance.

Sunaina chooses to do some **participatory action research** to help a group of British Asian women who speak little English to cope better with their respective disabilities. Specifically, she aims to study the effect of a new community outreach initiative designed to encourage these women to take up local rehabilitation opportunities. Sunaina aims to interview each participant both prior to the project and after six months. In addition, she will run an ongoing group to offer support and to monitor their changing needs. After a period of four months, she hopes that the women themselves will take on the running of this group. Sunaina is concerned that the women should be active participants in the programme and research project and she aims to involve them as co-researchers.

depend fundamentally on which methodology is adopted. Here we have five researchers embarking on projects that involve interviewing six participants about how they live and cope with disability. However, the similarities end there. The five researchers all have different aims for their research and they depart in completely different directions to explore different areas. These different aims have impacts not only on how the interviews are carried out and analysed, but also on the way the researchers see both their role and the nature of their research. In other words, the researchers have made significantly different methodological choices. Difficult ontological and epistemological concepts such as 'realism' and 'relativism' will be explained further in the next section. For now, just ride with the message of contrasting methodologies. Table 2.1 shows how the five case studies break down in terms of locating their respective methodologies, philosophies (epistemology and theory) and methods.

Table 2.1 Methodologies, philosophies and methods of the case studies

Name	Methodology	Philosophy Ontology/ epistemology	Theory	Method (data collection/ analysis)
Niall	Grounded theory	Realist, postpositivist	Less relevant – focus instead on published empirical work	Interview/ constant comparative method
Julie	Phenomenology	Critical realist, interpretivist	Ideas from work of Merleau-Ponty and other phenomenologists	Interview/ existential hermeneutic analysis
Masha	Discourse analysis	Relativist, post-structuralist	Ideas from work of Foucault and other sociologists	Interview/ Foucauldian discourse analysis
Johnson	Ethnography	Relativist, constructivist–interpretivist	Ideas stemming from anthropology and cultural studies	Interviews, participant observation/ ethnographic thematic analysis
Sunaina	Participatory action research	Realist, postpostivist	Less relevant – focus instead on published empirical work	Interviews, focus groups and questionnaires/ thematic and statistical analysis

Faced with competing methodologies, how do we choose? Often it comes down to practicalities like when a supervisor guides you in a particular direction. However, your preferences count too. You have to adopt a methodology to which you can relate. To identify and clarify your preferences, you might find it useful to reflect on your values, beliefs and interests; your goals; your resources and opportunities; your skills and knowledge; and any academic/disciplinary demands that influence you.

Returning to the case examples in Box 2.1, Niall chose a study that suited his natural science background and values. He wanted a research method that was more objective and clearly anchored in empirical data. Julie has a mental health background and she was interested in the personal and emotional aspects of her participants' experience. Masha believes in the power of societal factors to influence individuals' experience and she wanted a methodology to reflect this position. Johnson is a manager of a unit and he hoped to learn something about how the culture of a unit can be a positive influence. As a British Asian herself, Sunaina wanted to make a practical difference in, and for, her community. The next section continues this discussion of the link between methodology and method.

METHODOLOGY TO GUIDE METHODS

While all the people in Box 2.1 chose to do interviews, the techniques they used to collect their data would have differed. Niall and Sunaina probably used semi-structured interviews, while Julie, Masha and Johnson would have opted for less structured approaches. Their methods of actually carrying out their analyses will have diverged too (see Table 2.1): Niall would have used a constant comparative method to develop his grounded theory. Julie would have engaged in existential analysis, while Masha would have carried out a Foucauldian discourse analysis and Johnson an ethnographic analysis. Sunaina would have done a thematic content analysis of both her interviews and the group along with more quantitative statistical analysis of other data. Being clear about methodology would have helped these researchers to decide the most appropriate research methods (techniques and procedures) to use.

You'll read more about methods for data collection and analysis in Chapter 3. In the meantime, I'd just like to highlight two points about the relationship of methods to methodology. First, it is important to follow a coherent route, ensuring that your methods fit your methodology. There are natural affinities between methods and methodology, with the choice of data collection methods generally following from the choice of methodology. In ethnography, for instance, researchers do fieldwork that requires them to engage in participant observation (perhaps in combination with formal interviews and the reading of documents). A discourse analytic study requires a 'text' (some analysts are content to use interviews, while others prefer naturally occurring texts culled from conversations, media resources or published documents). A phenomenological researcher usually draws on interviews or other personal written accounts. Participatory action research tends to rely on focus groups or interview data, perhaps in combination with a survey or two. Other methodologies employ their own specific techniques. For instance, personal construct methodology utilises repertory grid technique.

Secondly, it is useful to be aware of the debates that exist within particular methodologies about the best methods to collect and analyse data. Within broad methodologies there are significantly different variants and with these come debates about the best way to apply methods. There are, for instance, different – though overlapping – versions of phenomenology. Descriptive phenomenologists inspired by Husserlian ideas (Giorgi and Giorgi, 2003) would attempt to study 'essences of phenomena as they appear in consciousness' (i.e. they take a more essentialist position). In contrast, hermeneutic researchers following Heidegger prefer to focus on 'existential dimensions' (Ashworth, 2003), exploring a person's sense of self, space, time, embodiment and relations with others in a less essentialist way. In interpretative phenomenological analysis (IPA) (Smith and Osborn, 2003) we find another hermeneutic variant – one that is more idiographic in intent (concerned with individual case studies), focused as it is on the individual's cognitive, linguistic, affective and physical being.

To emphasise this point further, consider the lesson learned by one of my students who attempted a discourse analytic study. She transcribed her data in a particular style and then found herself handicapped when she attempted her analysis. She needed to choose early on whether she wanted to do a Foucauldian analysis (which explores the ways in which discourse constructs subjectivity, selfhood and power relations) or detailed conversation analysis reading (examining the performative qualities of discourse). Foucauldian analysis (see Parker, 1992) examines how objects/subjects are constructed through discourse: for instance, what it is like to be positioned as 'criminally insane'. The latter method, seen in the work of Potter (1997), among others, is primarily concerned with how people use their everyday talk to achieve interpersonal objectives, such as attributing blame, justifying actions or disclaiming undesirable identities. My student needed to recognise that her initial data collection suggested a particular philosophical path and, once she had embarked on it, it would be difficult to change midstream.

In practice, our choice of data collection and analysis methods is invariably constrained by the resources we have available and by what is practical given the timeframe. We have to be pragmatic and sometimes compromises need to be made. Qualitative researchers commonly use interviews, for example, as these are relatively easy to arrange, while fieldwork involving participant observation can be difficult to set up and extremely time consuming. Master's level students may be well advised to confine themselves to a few basic interviews. Sometimes, the choices are guided by our participants. They may not want to be observed, or they may not have the verbal skills to cope with an interview. Alternative methods then need to be found. However, whatever the constraints, the methods must fit the chosen methodologies.

It is not always necessary for methods to follow rigidly from particular methologies – there is some flexibility to combine approaches. Nevertheless, it is essential to adopt a coherent, consistent route. Holloway and Todres (2003, p. 355) advise researchers that 'unreflective and undisciplined eclecticism might be avoided, not necessarily by settling on one approach as an exclusive commitment but by applying and making explicit an epistemological position that can coherently underpin its empirical claims.' (See Holloway and Todres (2003) for an analysis of points of consistency and flexibility between three methodologies.) Just what 'making explicit an epistemological position' means is explained in the next section.

CHOOSING YOUR PHILOSOPHICAL POSITION

PHILOSOPHICAL CHOICES

All research draws on ideas from particular research philosophies (also called 'paradigms'), albeit in sometimes unrecognised and taken-for-granted ways. Denzin and Lincoln (1994), for instance, recognise four 'world views': positivist and postpositivist; constructivist–interpretive; critical (Marxist, emancipatory); and feminist–poststructural. In this typology **positivists** and **postpositivists** work within objective, realist approaches (for instance using experimental and survey methods). In Box 2.1, Niall's approach fits this category. In contrast, the **constructivist–interpretive** paradigm, seen most commonly in ethnographic, phenomenological and narrative research – like in Julie's and Johnson's projects – takes a more naturalistic, relativist stance that recognises multiple meanings and subjective realities. The **critical** paradigm, found in politically oriented emancipatory research such as Sunaina's, privileges a materialist–realism (the idea that people are structured or shaped by socioeconomic relations) and naturalistic, subjectivist methodologies. The **feminist–poststructuralist** view emphasises problems with social texts and their inability ever to represent the world: an example is the social constructionist goal of deconstructing the language used in a particular instance and exploring its rhetorical functions. Masha's research fits this category.

Confronting such typologies, with their dense, abstract philosophical language, is daunting for most of us. For this reason, some researchers prefer to avoid grappling with these ideas altogether, seeing them as excessively academic territory that they don't need to articulate in their work. In reality, however, all research is inevitably going to be located somewhere, even if researchers don't acknowledge this. Further, I'd argue that difficulty and challenge are part of any worthwhile adventure. If your research is going to have coherence, credibility and depth, you need to venture at least a few steps into paradigm territory. And while words such as 'epistemology' are initially offputting, it's worth getting to grips with what they mean. To quote one student of mine:

> The first few months of my research I was in a complete fog. Words like epistemology did my head in. But suddenly it all clicked. It made sense! I realised these ideas were fundamental and I had been dealing with epistemology even when I didn't know it. (Personal communication)

I would argue further that a large part of the interest and enjoyment of research comes from grappling with the different ideas involved and debating them in the wider academic community. Researchers employing different research traditions often engage in intense debate about their competing philosophical positions! Positivists lock horns with interpretivists; realists with relativists; structuralists with functionalists; essentialists with constructionists; humanists with critical theorists, and so forth. This debate is part of the context of your research as well as how your research will be evaluated by others. The diversity of philosophies characterises qualitative research today – though qualitative researchers tend to unite immediately, of course, when challenged by quantitative researchers!

GETTING TO GRIPS WITH 'EPISTEMOLOGY'

Epistemology is concerned with the theory of knowledge and the role of science. It questions what, and how, we know things. Philosophers use it to look at the way we think about the nature of the social world and of our being (i.e. our ontology). In research terms, our epistemology defines how we conceptualise the nature and status of our research enterprise. To identify our own epistemological commitment we pose such questions as: What understanding am I aiming for? What kind of knowledge can I possibly gain? How do I understand the role of the researcher? These questions are fundamental to our research choices and it is well worth looking at them in more detail.

What Understanding Am I Aiming For?

One way of identifying the aims of our research is ask whether it falls into the positivist or interpretivist tradition. Positivists aim for 'truth', while interpretivists explore multiple meanings and interpretations. Positivists are optimistic about the possibility of gaining true knowledge about the 'real' world, which is seen to exist independently of our perceptions of it. Interpretivists, on the other hand, assert the impossibility of capturing 'truth' because truth is relative: there is not one 'reality', they argue, but many; what is true for you may not be true for me – it all depends on our perspective. Different people identify different realities as a result of 'construction and negotiation deeply embedded in culture' (Bruner, 1990, pp. 24–5). Box 2.2 describes each of these positions in more detail.

From the description in Box 2.2, you can see that quantitative research (based on the tenets of natural science) rests on positivist epistemological assumptions, while qualitative research tends towards interpretivism. That divide is just the starting point, however. Of the numerous qualitative research methodologies, some rest on assumptions close to those of positivism, while others are more thoroughly interpretivist. Even then, within particular methodologies, there can be differences. Grounded theory, for instance, is usually represented as being 'postpositivist'.

However, there are social constructionist versions which have an 'interpretivist' flavour (e.g. Charmaz, 1994).

> ### Box 2.2   Positivism versus interpretivism
>
> **Positivist** epistemology argues that the goal of research is object-
> ive knowledge gained through the labours of the researcher as
> an impartial, 'outside' observer. The 'neutral' scientist who sets out
> to record behaviours and discover some general patterns or the-
> ories about behaviour is adopting a positivist approach. Here the
> scientist is assuming that there is a relatively straightforward rela-
> tionship between the world (objects/events) and our perceptions
> and understanding of it. The scientist believes it is possible, at least
> to a reasonable degree, to describe and explain what is going on
> in the world.
>
> **Interpretivist** epistemology, in contrast, draws attention to the
> way our perceptions and experiences are socially, culturally, his-
> torically and linguistically produced. It argues that our situated-
> ness 'determines' our understanding. Thus, two researchers
> studying the same phenomenon may well interpret and under-
> stand that phenomenon differently. Interpretivist researchers
> argue that it is impossible to be objective, as the researcher's iden-
> tity and standpoint shape the research process and findings in a
> fundamental way. The interpretivist researcher recognises that
> they are part of the world they are studying, rather than external
> to it. Any understanding they gain from research informs them
> simultaneously about the object of study and about their own pre-
> occupations, expectations and cultural traditions. For the inter-
> pretivist researcher, understandings gained from research remain
> provisional, partial and entirely dependent on context.

What Kind of Knowledge Can I Possibly Gain?

Linked to the positivist–interpretivist debate is the one between realists and relativists concerning ontology (understandings about the
nature of the world). The **realist** position maintains that the world is
made up of structures and objects that have cause–effect relationships
with each other. Phenomena are seen to be made up of essential structures that can be identified and described. The aim is to study and
measure that real world 'out there'. For instance, realists argue that illnesses are objectively real and that we need to examine their effects

on people. The **relativist** position, in contrast, emphasises the diversity of interpretations that can be applied. While an illness may be 'real', the meanings that individual people have about the illness, in terms of how they experience it and also how it is understood from the outside, are multiple (i.e. relative and open to considerable variation). An extreme relativist position wouldn't even accept the 'reality' of an illness. If there were no words for an illness, they'd say, we wouldn't be aware of it and see it as troublesome. In this way, relativists argue that all experience is relative, being mediated, therefore constructed, through language. In between the two poles of realism and relativism is a position variously called '**critical realist**' (Guba and Lincoln, 1994), 'subtle realist' (Seale, 1999) or 'new realist' (Wetherell and Still, 1996). Here researchers tend to be pragmatic. They consider meanings to be fluid, while accepting that participants' stories of having an illness do reflect something of their subjective perceptions of their experience (if not their actual experience).

As qualitative researchers, we view our epistemology as broadly interpretivist, but vary considerably on where we place ourselves on the realism–relativism continuum. Phenomenologists usually adopt realist or critical realist positions, as they seek to capture, as closely as possible, the way in which a phenomenon is experienced and its essential structures. Discourse analytic researchers, in contrast, often view texts, such as interview transcripts, as simply one version obtained in a specific social context. While the text can be examined for broader social and cultural meanings, any knowledge gained from the data is seen as relative: contingent, partial, emergent and co-constructed.

How Do I Understand the Role of the Researcher?

All qualitative research methodologies recognise, at least to some degree, that the researcher is implicated in the research process. They agree that the researcher is a central figure who influences the collection, selection and interpretation of data and that our prior experience and understandings effect how we construct what we see. Qualitative researchers recognise that our behaviour, and the relationships we have with our participants, have an impact on our participants' responses, and hence the findings we obtain. Research is generally viewed as co-constituted: a joint product of the participants, the researcher and their relationship. Because meanings are negotiated within particular social contexts, other researchers are likely to unfold different stories (Finlay, 2002).

In order to develop self-awareness of these inter-subjective dynamics, qualitative researchers usually engage in **reflexivity**. This involves critical self-reflection, focusing on the ways a researcher's social background, assumptions, positioning and behaviour affect the research process. How this reflexive analysis is done, however, varies between researchers from different traditions. In one tradition, 'doing reflexivity' may mean providing a transparent methodological account, while in another it may involve exploring the dynamics between researcher and researched. Some researchers use reflexivity to examine the power of the researcher critically, while others use it to deconstruct pretences of established meanings. (See Finlay, 2003 for a review.)

The role of the researcher, then, is open to considerable debate. Different methodologies see the researcher as either being the 'author' or the 'witness' of their research findings (Willig, 2001). In grounded theory, the researcher's role is often viewed as that of a witness who faithfully records what the participant is saying and what is going on. Here, the researcher aims to be neutral and to avoid importing biases or assumptions into the analysis. The researcher's role is to represent, in as systematic a way as possible, the participants' world and perspective. With reference to fieldwork, for example, Morse recommends:

> The researcher should enter the setting as a 'stranger'. If the researcher is already familiar with the setting in a nonresearch capacity, then special precautions must be taken to avoid threats to validity (e.g. bias) . . . Familiarity with the setting or previous acquaintance with the participants dulls the researcher's ability to view the setting with the sensitivity one would have when seeing it for the first time. (Morse, 1993, p. 27)

In contrast, when discourse analysts emphasise the constructive and functional nature of language, they acknowledge that they are the authors of their research, playing an active role in the construction of their findings. They take seriously the need to be reflexively aware of the problematic status of their knowledge claims and the discourses used to construct them. From his social constructionist perspective, for instance, Gough (1999) explores his use of humour to breach the 'detached researcher' stance. In the following extract, Gough (called Bren) uses his data to examine reflexively his sense of discomfort on somehow 'colluding with the lads' – his participants. The subsequent analysis provided valuable data for his broader critique of 'men, masculinities and discourse'.

> Jack – . . . people look to label because it makes them feel safer . . . they think they know where they stand and they can control, but it's a lot more complex . . .

Bren – Psychologists are the worst offenders! [group laughter]

Jack – Yeah . . .

Glen – the media, the *Guardian* and psychologists on Channel 4! [group laughter].

I suppose the use of humour helps to suggest the illusion of 'normal' conversation, with the researcher temporarily colluding as one of the 'lads', albeit in this case one limited to one-line questions and interjections. This particular example could indicate a degree of self-deprecation, perhaps in an effort to reduce power differentials, or perhaps more likely, to create distance between myself and (the maligned) psychologists, hence appearing liberal or sophisticated (either way attempting to endear myself to the participants). Perhaps such occasional contributions give the impression of participation, thus rendering temporarily the otherwise peculiar position of polite interrogator less salient. It is also possible that humour is attempted as a defense in the light of anxiety or discomfort around my 'difference' (as researcher, tutor, outsider) and 'using' the participants for data. (Gough, 2003)

Taking a middle position, psychodynamic researchers could be said to act as both witness (in seeking to represent participants' experience) and author (in the way they produce interpretations). They, too, take seriously the need to examine reflexively their own responses to become aware of the emotional investment they have in the research. In her work on the police, Hunt (1989) identifies how her status as an unwanted female outsider raised a number of unconscious personal issues that then had an impact on the research relationship:

Positive oedipal wishes also appeared to be mobilized in the fieldwork encounter. The resultant anxieties were increased because of the proportion of men to women in the police organization and the way in which policemen sexualized so many encounters . . . The fact that I knew more about their work world than their wives also may have heightened anxiety because it implied closeness to subjects. By partly defeminizing myself through the adoption of a liminal gender role, I avoided a conflictual oedipal victory. That the police represented forbidden objects of sexual desire was revealed in dreams and slips of the tongue . . . the intended sentence 'Jim's a good cop' came out instead 'Jim's a good cock'. In those words, I revealed my sexual interest in a category of men who were forbidden as a result of their status as research subjects. In that way, they resembled incestuous objects. (Hunt, 1989, p. 40)

So far in this section you have seen that what we understand and expect from research depends on our philosophical commitments and our epistemological stance as researchers. It also depends on what theoretical perspectives we bring to bear – the focus of the next section.

CHOOSING YOUR THEORETICAL PERSPECTIVE

There are myriad possible theoretical perspectives that qualitative researchers can embrace: social constructionism, structuralism, feminism, critical theory, phenomenology, humanism, symbolic interactionism, psychodynamic theory, personal construct theory – the list goes on.

These are not just isolated theories. They determine the course of the research and the quality or style of the findings. They also usually link back to particular methodologies and philosophies (for instance, the way Masha in Box 2.1 chose to do a 'Foucauldian' discourse analysis).

The powerful determining role of theory can be shown in the following example of a narrative analysis research (Finlay, 2004). Here, I offer two contrasting analyses of one man's (Kenny's) narrative of his journey towards finding a new occupational identity after experiencing mental health problems. I show that, depending on the perspective adopted, research can focus on different aspects of the story and reach different kinds of understanding. Boxes 2.3 and 2.4 describe briefly what these contrasting 'takes' look like. From a phenomenological perspective, for instance, the focus is on Kenny's subjective experience of his illness. By way of contrast, a social constructionist approach concentrates on how Kenny's story was told and 'performed'. In other words, simply listening to a person's story is only one part of the picture. 'Much depends on how we theoretically frame and reflexively analyse the narrative. The self-sufficiency of narratives . . . needs to be challenged' (Finlay, 2004, p. 480).

The two examples in Boxes 2.3 and 2.4 demonstrate how important it is to understand what theoretical perspective we're employing. Returning to the mapping metaphor, theory is our starting point and offers us choices between routes.

Sometimes one's own personal and research theoretical perspectives collide and can result in possible confusions or contradictory impulses. These need to be worked through. Here, for example, Willott (1998, p. 183) reflexively examines the individual, social-political and research implications of being a feminist researcher researching men:

> There is a tension between being a researcher and being a feminist. As a feminist I want to see a change in the patriarchal relations between men and women. I would like this change to extend to my relationships with

---

Box 2.3   A phenomenological account of Kenny's experience

Locking himself in his bedroom, he hides from a suddenly threatening world in a desperate attempt to be safe, protecting both himself and others. We catch a glimpse of his aloneness and terror as he struggles to understand what is happening to him. As his feelings go out of control, he loses control over himself and his life. His relationships with both himself and others are anxiety provoking, a feeling experienced all the more acutely as it is alien to his previously habitual way of being. The change in his 'being-in-the-world' (Heidegger, 1927/1962) – his altered consciousness and existence – is confusing and frightening. Past aims and projects have been derailed while the future becomes profoundly uncertain and bleak.

Then we hear of Kenny's journey of self-discovery and how he confronts and surmounts barriers of increasing challenge. Being able to 'kick down' each new hurdle successfully empowers Kenny and gives him more confidence. He describes some of the self-help strategies that have helped him cope. Through various metaphors, he talks of climbing up the ladder out of the pit and chipping away at the concrete block to find his confidence. We gain the sense of how he has motivated himself through his journey out of his mental health problems. In the end he is reconciled to letting his previous occupational identity go. (Finlay, 2004, p. 478)

---

the research participants, but found it difficult to challenge directly. As a researcher I was careful to nurture relationships, to avoid stepping over invisible lines in which these relationships might be jeopardized, and to 'enter sympathetically into the alien and possibly repugnant perspectives of rival thinkers'.

A more personal example is when, in my own PhD research on the life world of the occupational therapist (Finlay, 1998), I struggled with how to incorporate my feminist, social constructionist leanings into my phenomenological method. How was I to reconcile my socially oriented, relativist beliefs with the apparently individualistic, essentialist understandings (to say nothing of Heidegger's fascism) embedded in much of the phenomenological literature? In the end, I accepted that my 'choices' inevitably closed off some doors while opening others. It just took me a while to work out which doors I wanted to open!

Box 2.4   A social constructionist view of Kenny's 'performance'

As Riessman (2003, p. 8) noted: 'Individuals negotiate how they want to be known in the stories they develop collaboratively with their audiences . . . Social actors shape their lives retrospectively for particular audiences.' Here, Riessman (2003) is drawing on Goffman's (1959) celebrated dramaturgical metaphor, which showed how people 'perform' desirable selves to preserve 'face' in difficult situations, such as explaining, and coping with chronic illness. In this reading, identities are socially situated and accomplished with an audience in mind. The world can be likened to a stage and our narratives part of the show.

Kenny's performance can also be understood as a way of 'doing' masculinity (Edley, 2002). His struggle to respect himself through finding a work role needs to be seen in the context of the stigma arising in his working class community from being an unemployed man who is not fulfilling his family breadwinner role. Through his narrative performance focused on returning to work and becoming an 'iceman' he reasserts his preferred masculine identity. As Bourdieu and others have noted, 'narratives about the most "personal" . . . articulate the deepest structures of the social world' (Bourdieu *et al.*, 1993, cited in Riessman, 2003, p. 24). (Finlay, 2004, p. 478)

To summarise: In the last two sections, I've tried to show how philosophy and theory offer us a lens through which we can view our participants and the research process. They help us know how to approach our research and what to look for. They give us tools to analyse our data and assess the impact of our relationships with participants. The different philosophies and theories offer competing accounts, make claims as to legitimate knowledge and suggest divergent methodological routes. We need to be clear about which qualitative routes we are choosing.

FINAL REFLECTIONS

This chapter as a whole has sought to show the importance of methodology to research and to map some of the methodological paths confronting us when we embark on our qualitative research adventure. I have tried to demonstrate the profound influence of philosophy and theoretical ideas, both in terms of how we understand the nature of our journey and how we apply our methods.

To my mind, the researcher who adopts a particular method (say, interviewing) with the vague idea of doing 'qualitative analysis' is on dodgy ground from the very outset. I've had students come to me having already collected potentially valuable data, who now bemoan the fact that they don't know what to do with it. Had they started thinking about methodology earlier, they would have known what to do. In fact, they may have collected different data in the first place!

There are always difficult choices to make. Awareness that there are competing perspectives and alternative approaches acts as a continuing – and constructive – travel companion in our quest for knowledge.

That much enthusiastic – and sometimes vociferous – debate takes place between proponents of the different versions can be confusing for novice researchers trying to work out what they're trying to do. To the outsider this academic 'infighting' can seem obscure and pretentious. There are insiders, too, who oppose the splits and seek reconciliation and synthesis. Wetherell (1998), in specific reference to discourse analysis, argues that having such divisions of labour is counterproductive. Rather than regarding variants as mutually exclusive, researchers should be able to utilise the diversity of tools they offer pragmatically. If you adopt this approach, however, remember to ensure that epistemological and theoretical common ground can be established and that there can be no fundamental incompatibilities.

As researchers we need to decide the extent we are going to engage in these debates. At least, we should be able to acknowledge that we're wedded to a specific variant or are perhaps applying a method more loosely than is usual. At Master's level research, it may not be necessary to be precise. It might be sufficient to say, for instance, that you are simply going to do a 'grounded theory study using the constant comparative method'. You probably won't be required to sort out the subtleties of whether you are following the original ideas of Glaser and Strauss (1967) or later variants such as using the step-by-step guides (Strauss and Corbin, 1990) or less prescriptive versions (Glaser, 1992). PhD level research, however, is likely to require you to show that you understand the contested nature of analytic methods. It is likely that you will be encouraged to be clearer about your methodological commitments. Indeed, you might even be inspired to invent your own original methodology!

You will understand by now that there are no simple, comprehensive and clear-cut maps for methodology. The terrain, whichever way you look at it, is difficult and messy. Theory doesn't always translate well into practice. Far from being able to root our research firmly in theoretical principles, we may make decisions on pragmatic grounds. Qualitative research rarely progresses smoothly: even when we're confident we know where we're going, we can lose our way. We might start down one route only to confront a dead end and have to backtrack in search of a new way forward. We can also be torn in different ways, tempted by the promise of other routes. Constrained by time, resources and perhaps our own limited skills, we might be forced to take potentially risky shortcuts.

Nevertheless, having some kind of map provides support and guidance along the way. At the very least it should help explain why you may be lost! There are no easy or self-evident outcomes to our research adventure – but if we set off without first sorting out in our minds the nature of our journey, then our research may well prove muddled, inconclusive and of limited value. Being clear about the nature and purpose of our research journey will, at least, set us off in the right direction.

REFERENCES

Ashworth, P. (2003) 'An approach to phenomenological psychology: The contingencies of the lifeworld', *Journal of Phenomenological Psychology*, 34(2): 145–56.

Bourdieu, P., Accardo, A., Balazs, G., Beaud, S. *et al.* (1993) *The Weight of the World: Social Suffering in Contemporary Society* (trans. P.P. Ferguson *et al.*), Stanford, CA: Stanford University Press.

Bruner, J. (1990) *Acts of Meaning*, Cambridge, MA: Harvard University Press.

Charmaz, K. (1994) 'Experiencing chronic illness', in Albrecht, G.L., Fitzpatrick, R. and Scrimshaw, S.C. (eds), *The Handbook of Social Studies in Health and Medicine*, London: Sage.

Denzin, N.K. and Lincoln, Y.S. (1994) 'Introduction: Entering the field of qualitative research', in Denzin, N.K. and Lincoln, Y.S. (eds), *Handbook of Qualitative Research*, Thousand Oaks, CA: Sage Publications.

Edley, N. (2002) 'The loner, the walk and the beast within: Narrative fragments in the construction of masculinity', in Patterson, W. (ed.), *Strategic Narrative: New Perspectives on the Power of Personal and Cultural Stories*, Lanham, MD: Lexington Books.

Finlay, L. (1998) 'The life world of the occupational therapist: Meaning and motive in an uncertain world', unpublished PhD thesis, Milton Keynes: The Open University.

Finlay, L. (2002) 'Negotiating the swamp: The opportunity and challenge of reflexivity in research practice', *Qualitative Research*, 2(2): 209–30.

Finlay, L. (2003) 'The reflexive journey: Mapping multiple routes', in Finlay, L. and Gough, B. (eds), *Reflexivity: A Practical Guide for Researchers in Health and Social Sciences*, Oxford: Blackwell Science.

Finlay, L. (2004) 'From "gibbering idiot" to "iceman", Kenny's story: A critical analysis of an occupational narrative', *British Journal of Occupational Therapy*, 67(11): 474–80.

Giorgi, A. and Giorgi, B. (2003) 'Phenomenology', in Smith, J.A. (ed.), *Qualitative Psychology: A Practical Guide to Research Methods*, London: Sage.

Glaser, B.G. (1992) *Emergence vs Forcing: Basics of Grounded Theory Analysis*, Mill Valley, CA: Sociology Press.

Glaser, B.G. and Strauss, A.L. (1967) *The Discovery of Grounded Theory*, Chicago: Aldine.

Goffman, E. (1959) *The Presentation of Self in Everyday Life*, New York: Penguin.

Gough, B. (1999) 'Subject positions within discourse analysis: Some reflexive dilemmas', paper given at International Human Science Conference, July 26–29, Sheffield.

Gough, B. (2003) 'Shifting research positions during a group interview study: A reflexive analysis and re-view', in Finlay, L. and Gough, B. (eds), *Reflexivity: A Practical Guide for Researchers in Health and Social Sciences*, Oxford: Blackwell Science.

Guba, E.G. and Lincoln, Y.S. (1994) 'Competing paradigms in qualitative research', in Denzin, N.K. and Lincoln, Y.S. (eds), *Handbook of Qualitative Research*, Thousand Oaks: Sage.

Heidegger, M. (1927/1962) *Being and Time* (trans. J. Macquarrie and E. Robinson), Oxford: Basil Blackwell.

Holloway, I. and Todres, L. (2003) 'The status of method: Flexibility, consistency and coherence', *Qualitative Research* 3(3): 345–57.

Hunt, J.C. (1989) 'Psychoanalytic aspects of fieldwork', *Qualitative Research Methods*, 18, Beverly Hills, CA: Sage Publications.

Morse, J.M. (1993) '"Emerging from the data": The cognitive processes of analysis in qualitative inquiry', in Morse, J.M. (ed.), *Critical Issues in Qualitative Research Methods*, Thousand Oaks: Sage Publications.

Parker, I. (1992) *Discourse Dynamics: Critical Analysis for Social and Individual Psychology*, London: Routledge.

Potter, J. (1997) 'Discourse analysis as a way of analysing naturally occurring talk', in Silverman, D. (ed.), *Qualitative Research: Theory, Method and Practice*, London: Sage.

Riessman, C.K. (2003) 'Performing identities in illness narrative: Masculinity and multiple sclerosis', *Qualitative Research*, 3(1): 5–33.

Seale, C. (1999) *The Quality of Qualitative Research*, London: Sage Publications.

Smith, J.A. and Osborn, M. (2003) 'Interpretative phenomenological analysis', in Smith, J.A. (ed.), *Qualitative Psychology: A Practical Guide to Research Methods*, London: Sage Publications.

Strauss, A.L. and Corbin, J. (1990) *Basics of Qualitative Research: Grounded Theory Procedures and Techniques*, London: Sage Publications.

Wetherell, M. (1998) 'Positioning and interpretative repertoires: Conversation analysis and post-structuralism in dialogue', *Discourse and Society*, 9: 387–413.

Wetherell, M. and Still, A. (1996) 'Realism and relativism', in Sapsford, R. (ed.), *Issues for Social Psychology*, Buckingham: Open University Press.

Willig, C. (2001) *Introducing Qualitative Research in Psychology: Adventures in Theory and Method*, Buckingham: Open University Press.

Willott, S. (1998) 'An outsider within: A feminist doing research with men', in Henwood, K., Griffin, C. and Phoenix, A. (eds), *Standpoints and Differences*, London: Sage Publications.

3

Strategic Choices in Research Planning

BARBARA STEWARD

Research can often appear an uncertain activity, driven by external forces and taken off course by unexpected events. However, with good planning and clear understandings of the aims of the study, much of the process of research can be made more predictable and controllable. As researchers, we have to set out with a clear appreciation of how we conceptualise the study, what we intend to collect as appropriate data and within what conceptual frames it can be understood. Otherwise we can fall prey to endless searches for additional information, collecting so much data that meaningful analysis rarely emerges. Decisions about the aim of the study in relation to methodological theory have already been discussed. Here, I offer what I hope is a pragmatic approach to making choices about the research and following through a research method.

I will focus on seven key decisions:

- Choosing a topic.
- Gathering together support systems and resources.
- Locating and understanding existing knowledge.
- Framing the research question.
- Selecting the method of research data collection.
- Recruiting participants.
- Synthesising and analysing the data.

This is not an exclusive list, and other types and elements of decision trails will be described by authors in their critical appraisal of their own

Qualitative Research for Allied Health Professionals: Challenging Choices. Edited by Linda Finlay and Claire Ballinger. Copyright 2006 by John Wiley & Sons Ltd. ISBN 0-470-01963-8.

research projects. Ethical considerations, of central importance to all research, will be discussed separately in Chapter 4.

CHOOSING A TOPIC

When embarking on research, the first step is to ask yourself a series of questions. Why do you want to do this study, now, on this particular topic? Why do you want to do it with these people, in this way, over this period of time and in this location? What results do you anticipate? This list indicates the wide range of key decisions that have to be made early in the research process. Research may be driven by personal, professional or academic goals, which will influence its structure and timescale. Whatever your motivations, you need to consider closely the available resources, your existing knowledge and beliefs, and what you expect to be the outcomes of the study. Research should not be seen as an intrinsically noble, heroic or laudable endeavour, but rather as a fascinating, and challenging, way to develop personal and professional understanding.

The first choice you need to make in the research process is to decide what captures your imagination and 'turns you on'. While experienced researchers may have a clear career pathway that determines the topics they will investigate, Bogdan and Biklen (1998) note that for the novice researcher 'the question of what to study is more perplexing' (1998, p. 59). A topic may emerge from a clinical observation or problem. It may arise from recognising a gap in knowledge and a desire to explore an unknown. Because our beliefs and motives inform our initial choices of what to study, we need to recognise this from the very outset. Such transparency helps us identify sources of potential 'bias' and prejudice. I would argue that it is impossible to begin a research project of special personal interest without having already formed some opinions about its nature and implications. These personal interests cannot be quarantined merely by identifying them as a possible problem and hoping thereby to free all other choices from their effects. The interests have to be actively and reflexively worked through. Even the concept of 'bias' could be usefully interrogated. Many qualitative researchers, for instance, would reject the concept as it suggests a deviation from a 'real' or proper route.

Our personal perspectives will always influence how we actually set about collecting, synthesising and analysing the data. As researchers, we need to make our standpoint clear through a process of reflexivity

(Finlay and Gough, 2003; Oakley, 1981). Our own 'voice' as the researcher needs to be heard throughout in discussions of how the topic is selected, investigated and analysed and in terms of where we stand in relation to the topic, the study context and the key informants. Through reflexivity we can also examine how our beliefs and values change as a result of carrying out the research.

Whatever the choice of topic, it should be something that fascinates and excites. If it fails to generate enthusiasm and curiosity, a project will become like the burden of Sisyphus: an endless and hopeless labour.

GATHERING TOGETHER SUPPORT SYSTEMS AND RESOURCES

Following on the heels of the choice of research topic are decisions about how the project will be supervised and managed. Selecting a supervisor, research panel members, co-researcher and consultants requires careful consideration of their role and responsibilities and how they will help steer your research or contribute to data analysis. Your choice of methodology will clarify the selection process. To avoid later confusion or conflict, it is advisable to negotiate what is expected of supervisors or co-researchers at an early stage. In my own case, I needed a supervisor who could span the disciplines of sociology, psychology, business and health. A lengthy process ensued in which I held discussions with various possible supervisors and sought to establish where our interests and attitudes coincided. Eventually I selected medical sociology as my 'home'.

Early decisions also have to be made on the availability of both internal and external resources. What time and commitment can you make to the study? What skills might you need to acquire? External resources such as computer hardware and software, IT support, study space, library access and peer support require considerable planning. Good logistics can save time and grief later. In addition, you need to consider resources and constraints attached to any funding you may receive. In my case, I had to conform to limitations placed by the agency funding my research on the publication and presentation of my findings. Each funding agency will have some rules of engagement tied to acceptance of the awards it makes. As researchers, we have to decide whether we can live with possible external constraints. We also need to consider whether the link between our research and public or private funds may reduce the independence of our research in the eyes of others.

LOCATING AND UNDERSTANDING
EXISTING KNOWLEDGE

A literature review is a key element of any research. It serves a range
of functions: to establish whether similar research has already been
undertaken; to identify how the topic has already been framed; and to
see how key issues have been defined or conceptualised. There is a need
to review the evidence at some stage, whether this precedes or follows
the data collection and preliminary analysis. Although we may want to
avoid having our ideas shaped too much by others in advance, some
preliminary reading of the literature is usually needed to avoid dupli-
cation of research effort.

A literature review has five key purposes:

1. To offer a thorough **overview of the topic**, to provide a broad
    context that will synthesise the evidence about what is known
    about the topic, how these ideas have been developed, what
    controversies exist, what are the key ideas and who are the key
    theorists.
2. To offer specific **details about the research topic**, to define terms,
    debate contested meanings and position key research within epis-
    temological frames.
3. To **appraise the evidence** critically, offering a methodical evalua-
    tion of the quality of the data. The review should analyse the quality
    and content of the existing evidence. The review should offer a bal-
    anced account of the evidence, not one side that supports your own
    or a particular viewpoint.
4. To **justify the need for the current research**, identifying gaps in the
    evidence. This may include highlighting a special dimension of a
    topic that has yet to be explored, or a participant group whose
    experiences of an already researched topic have yet to be exam-
    ined. It should also justify the selected methodology and method.
5. To **develop a knowledge base** within which your own research find-
    ings will contribute new data and insights, and within which you
    will debate and critique your findings.

Reviews should include this synthesis, critical appraisal and analysis,
and the process needs to be fully explained and justified (Steward,
2004). While engaged in your literature review, it is important to keep
the purpose of the exercise at the forefront of your mind. One of your
aims is to help readers understand the evidence and the analysis you
build on its basis. You want them to comprehend the need for your

research and the basis on which you make your findings. If, as in a grounded theory approach, your main literature review search is undertaken after themes have emerged from the study, you need to carry readers with you. After all, they may well be expecting a more conventional, scientific report-style format.

It is possible to have problems satisfying the requirements of the funding body, ethics and research governance committees, who expect a proposal that describes and critiques the existing evidence. However, this may be at odds with your methodology, in which *a priori* assumptions are deliberately avoided because themes are expected to emerge from the process of the research. Such problems may be acute where committees approving research apply submission criteria more appropriate to quantitative studies. While qualitative research is now far more widely accepted, we need to write clear and precise proposals to indicate the more complex relationship that exists between analysis of published evidence and the new generation of working theories. Sometimes, however, the requirements of the awards panel may have to prevail and you may need to make compromises to avoid your proposal being rejected.

Literature reviewing is not a single enterprise but is continuous throughout the research as themes and working theories emerge. You might select formal appraisal methods and follow guides for the selection of databases, key words and inclusion and exclusion criteria (NHS CRD, 2001; Law *et al.*, 1998; Morse, 2003). Searches will often go beyond allied health or medical databases to include sources from other disciplines. In the case of my own study, the emergent themes took me to the literature on utopian philosophies, the sociology of time and human geography. Parochialism in relation to your review of literature should be avoided lest the richness of interdisciplinary theory and research is lost.

The critical appraisal of existing evidence poses problems. When we comment on the rigour of others' research, it is inappropriate and unprofessional to pillory other authors or simply rubbish their work. Our aim is to give a balanced and reasoned critique of their methodological strengths and weaknesses rather than simply to air our opinions.

A literature review is, in itself, a process of exploring and analysing secondary data. As such, it has parameters in the same way as does a primary research project. It cannot be done quickly. And, just like any research undertaking, it can be poorly done. Poor reviews, for example, could take the form of simple listings of citations, presented as strings of names in brackets. They could amount to little more than an annotated opinion piece. Or they could comprise a series of short descriptions of research papers located through computer search engines.

Overall, reviewing the literature requires us to make a series of choices relating to search, appraisal, synthesis and analysis. We need to consider what key words to use and employ dynamic relationships between them to expand or restrict our searches. Our aim is not only to select key words but also to interrogate their meaning and usage in different disciplines. Only on this basis can we challenge our own taken-for-granted understanding of meanings. A review is an eclectic mix of evidence through which we sift to identify themes, debates and controversies.

FRAMING THE RESEARCH QUESTION

The research question is the most important statement we have to make about the subject matter and the mode of investigation. It is also the most difficult. Key decisions have to be stated right at the very start of the study. The previous chapter identified the ease with which novice researchers often drift into method, deciding strategies for data collection without determining what they want to study, why and with what epistemological perspective.

The first problem is to select a well-defined topic of manageable size. Silverman (1993) recommends differentiating between social problems and research problems. Topics in the former category, such as health or unemployment, may well be too global, or lack sufficient focus for research purposes. Noting how new researchers tend to gravitate towards impossibly large research problems, Silverman (1993) says that the aim should be to say 'a lot about a little problem' (1993, p. 3).

There can be confusion about both the form and the purpose of the research question. It is the question that you, as the researcher, anticipate can be answered or at least discussed from the analysis of the data collected. This is not necessarily the same question that participants will be asked. Research questions pose the central question, which subsequently will be subdivided into subsidiary themes of investigation. In my own study the research question was: 'Do new forms of employment affect experiences of health and wellbeing?' The subsidiary questions were: 'What is telework in the eyes of those who say they are doing it?' and 'What is illness and sickness for those who define themselves as teleworkers?'

Beyond indicating the topic under study, the research question indicates a broad methodology and the purpose of the study. It should also indicate the form that the study will take. Punch (1998, p. 38) identifies five roles for the research question:

- To give direction and coherence to the project.
- To identify its boundaries.
- To provide a focus for the investigation.
- To offer a framework for writing up the project.
- To indicate what data will be needed to answer it.

Posing the question can present problems. To what extent can a research question be framed in advance of the study actually being carried out? Will research governance and ethics committees accept a research question that aims to explore uncharted territory with unpredictable outcomes? Can the question be framed to explain a method that involves emergent design and emergent themes? Framing the question involves the researcher in treading a careful line: that of defining the broad parameters of the study without making it too prescribed, or implying foreknowledge of what participants will think and say.

Returning to the examples offered in the previous chapter (Box 2.1), the research questions of Niall, Sunaina and Masha are subtly different. Although all are interested in the same topic, the question that each frames reflects the different methodologies they plan to utilise.

For Niall, the question that best reflects and represents his realist assumptions and his chosen grounded theory methodology might be:

> What coping mechanisms do people with disabilities adopt and what makes these effective?

Sunaina, whose interest lies in using a phenomenological approach to explore participants' life worlds, might frame her question thus:

> What is the everyday subjective experience of disability?

Masha, whose focus is on the way people narrate their experiences and the extent to which such narrations represent individual and cultural discourse, might frame her research question along the following lines:

> How do people tell their stories of disability and what does this suggest about how people construct and are constructed by social concepts of disability?

Some academic or funding bodies will expect research questions to identify aims and objectives. Yet predetermining outcomes in qualitative research may impose something of a straightjacket. Seale (1998) suggests that the research question and the choice of literature in the review should indicate whether the study aims to influence policy, practice or theory. When writing a proposal it may be advantageous to indicate in which of these domains you expect your research will have most influence. This is rather different to research questions predicting that new methods of treatment **will** be formulated or understanding patient perspectives **will** lead to better service delivery, and presupposes that analysis of the data can and will achieve this aim. While it is not incorrect to impose, top down, *a priori* concepts on qualitative data, results may be most productive when exploring the unknown and challenging the taken for granted.

The following research questions make predictions that could influence questions and observations at the interview stage, as well as the interpretation of the data:

- How do clients experience depression and how can their perceptions be used to improve existing home-based mental health care delivery?
- How successful is vocational rehabilitation in preparing service users for return to paid work following chronic illness?
- What aspects of a physiotherapy programme are considered by patients to be most effective in regaining full mobility?

Such questions suggest the researcher's agenda and predict that certain routes in data collection and analysis might be closed as a result.

More open-ended alternatives could be considered. For example:

- How do clients describe their experience of depression and what do they think might be ways to improve the choice and delivery of mental health support?
- What are the experiences of service users returning to work following discharge from vocational rehabilitation programmes and how do they account for success or failure?
- What do patients do in physiotherapy mobilisation sessions and how do they understand what they are instructed to do and evaluate its effectiveness?

Such changes alter not only expectations about the outcome of the research but also the methods used. We need to spend time thinking about, and debating with others, the focus of each study.

One thing is for sure: none of us begins research without beliefs, values and opinions. The very choice of research question reveals an interest in, and opinion about, the topic. It indicates where we stand in relation to the participants, be they data providers or research collaborators. Framing the research question is often the first stage of reflection. It enables us to think about the presumptions we bring to the topic and what we expect to achieve from the research. Reflecting on these issues by writing a reflective diary and sharing this with supervisors, co-researchers and research panels (which may include participants) may serve to clarify the research question further.

SELECTING THE METHOD OF RESEARCH DATA COLLECTION

A method is like a recipe. It explains and defines what will be done and in what manner. Unlike a recipe, however, it should be chosen for clear theoretical reasons. Methods are often chosen for pragmatic reasons. These run the risk of being inconsistent with the methodology and poorly grounded in theory. Data collection methods cannot be justified because they seem to be the easiest way forward or because time is limited. Researchers have to demonstrate that their choice of method and procedures offers the best way of answering their research question.

The research topic itself may well suggest which approach is appropriate for gathering data. In the case of the study into how clients describe their experience of depression and how they think mental health support might be improved, the research topic points to interviewing as the primary method of data collection. In contrast, the research question on what patients do in physiotherapy mobilisation sessions indicates that observation of patients' activities will play a central role.

Novice researchers tend to choose a method with which they feel comfortable or of which they have had some previous experience. Observation is often avoided because it poses special problems (for example, selective recording) as well as ethical issues such as intrusion. Choice of method is a challenge that has to be fully considered before any data collection is commenced. The method you choose needs to

- match the methodology;
- establish and justify the type and number of participants;

- offer a fair and full opportunity for participants to provide information relating to the research question;
- make overt the relationship between the researcher and the researched to all involved in the study and to subsequent readers of the project report;
- allow for the advance planning of data collection, recording and analysis;
- take into account issues of trustworthiness and validation.

Once a method is chosen, further decisions will need to be made. For example, if your method involves interviewing, you will have to decide whether to use structured, semi-structured or unstructured questioning. In observational studies, you would have to balance the relative merits of being a participant or nonparticipant observer. Each choice will have implications for your study and your analysis and subsequent theory building.

An example from my own work illustrates this point. I wanted participants to describe in their own words the lived experience of teleworking. To this end, I used an unstructured format for the initial part of the first interview. In the second part I picked up on themes and ideas that had already emerged and sought further information and, where necessary, clarification. In the second interview, however, I employed focused questioning, based on my preliminary analysis, to explore themes further. Many of my participants had described feeling uncomfortable with giving a rambling account and had told me that they preferred to give specific answers to focused questions. In the first interview they had provided individual narrative accounts that were relatively unshaped by my presuppositions, but that were influenced by their sense of discomfort and their inability to frame a spontaneous story with a coherent temporal or motivational thread. They perceptibly relaxed when I moved into asking them focused questions. However, this involved me imposing my structure and my preliminary analysis, and in the process the nuances of their spontaneous accounts were lost.

Subsequent chapters in this book will examine similar decisions about applying research methods. Each method has its own benefits, limitations and problems. Some of these can be predicted, while others will emerge in the course of the study. The important thing is to be able to provide a detailed account of the method used.

RECRUITING PARTICIPANTS

In studies using participants, the process of how to select, access, inform and retain research participants requires considerable thought. Sampling is a key issue, because it is impossible to know what everyone does or thinks in every situation at all times (Miles and Huberman, 1994). There is often confusion between sampling methods employed for quantitative research and those more appropriate for qualitative methods. Quantitative sampling involves probability sampling determined by the mathematical calculation of statistics. These calculate the sample size and identify a representative group from whom findings can be generalised back to the study population from which they have been drawn. Participants here would be randomly selected to ensure that they are a representative sample. In qualitative studies other factors determine the choice of participants. The process of recruitment varies with the stated purpose of the study. The variety – and complexity – of the available recruitment methods can easily overwhelm the researcher (Patton, 1987).

Decisions about whom to recruit for research rest in the first instance on whether the study is examining the views/behaviours of a homogeneous group or of a broad social spectrum. It is common for findings to describe the demographic characteristics of a group, but not explain whether such demographics are the result of design or chance. We need to be explicit about whether people are specialist informants, extreme cases and/or naïve subjects if sense is to be made of our findings. The choice of method – whether convenience, purposive or snowballing – needs to be coherent and fit with the methodology and method employed. Often participants are difficult to locate, and sometimes desperate measures may have to be undertaken to get people involved. In such cases, the whole research process appears to go off course. However, these events may indicate important issues about the people we are investigating, including their accessibility and their ability to be involved in research. We need to provide a transparent account of how we undertook the recruitment of participants. For example, were inducements or rewards offered? Were our participants recruited on the basis of invitation? Did they volunteer their involvement? Were they, however slightly, coerced into explaining their narratives or actions?

Recruiting participants is far from an exact science. In an attempt to rationalise the choice, some texts suggest ideal numbers and rather formal procedures geared to selecting the 'right' people (Crabtree and

Miller, 1992; Lincoln and Guba, 1985). Selection procedures involving purposeful, deviant, typical case, homogeneous or maximum variation or convenience sampling are available (Patton, 1987). Overall, the aim is to gather the type and number of participants likely to offer data relevant to the research question and appropriate to the chosen methodology.

In action research or feminist projects, the expectation is that participants will take on a greater role in planning, analysing and implementing the findings. Recruiting people who can work in a collaborative way, and commit time and effort to the study, may require a different type of selection process. Relating to participants is of increasing importance if you wish them to be involved in participant validation or co-construction of the data.

There are a number of key questions to consider when thinking about the recruitment of participants:

- How accessible do you think these particular participants will be?
- Are there any risks attached to their being involved?
- Do you expect them to offer spontaneous or considered opinions about the topic?
- Will they be involved in the formulation and/or the validation of your preliminary and final analyses?
- Will they be expected to have an extended relationship with the research project?
- If they are being selected as an idiosyncratic or extreme case, should they be informed about this?
- Are you intending to pay them for their participation? Or will they get involved on a strictly voluntary basis, with no payment offered? Might you offer to cover their expenses?

You might develop specific criteria of inclusion and exclusion to help identify appropriate informants or those who might be at particular risk through being a participant. You will need to consider whether you are unfairly eliminating people from the investigation because they are difficult to locate or tricky to interview. You may need to think about the implications of the over- or under-involvement of certain types of people, or of those with particular experiences or opinions.

Sample size is an equally important issue. Poor qualitative reports often conclude by noting that if only there had been more time to interview a larger number of participants, the results would have been better. Few grounded theory studies have the time and opportunity to adopt the notion of saturation fully (Sim and Wright, 2000), where people are interviewed until all the possible themes have been raised. While such an approach is irrelevant for other methodologies, each method requires us to calculate how many people we should and can involve in the study in order to maximise the trustworthiness of the research. It is considered unethical to recruit participants who are then not involved. Although you may anticipate attrition in the study, you cannot have a 'substitutes' bench' of surplus participants. If people drop out, you will have to recruit replacements – or accept (and explain) the implications of participants dropping out of the study.

Deciding on the number of participants for a qualitative study is a thorny issue. More does not mean better. A careful calculation needs to be made, and the choice justified on the basis of the study's method. For example, Sarah Dean, Sheila Payne and Jonathan Smith, in Chapter 10 of this book, used a purposive sample of nine patients with back pain for their interview-based study. Anne Killett (Chapter 12) describes the varying involvement of her initial 16 volunteers. Linda Finlay (Chapter 13) employed a case-study approach with one respondent, while Tanya Campbell-Breen and Fiona Poland (Chapter 11) located a number of participants using gatekeepers, selecting only six for detailed data analysis. I would suggest that no mathematical calculation can be applied to the number of participants for qualitative studies. However, the recruitment process, and the number of participants recruited, need to be fully explained and justified. In some cases, the recruitment process may need to be adjusted as the study progresses and new information is sought or explored. None of this may be helpful perhaps to new researchers hoping for a simple solution. But it does indicate the importance of making a choice of participants based on the methodology and method of your particular research venture.

SYNTHESISING AND ANALYSING THE DATA

Proposals and research reports often offer limited information about the analytical methods planned and employed. They may suggest vaguely that the researcher has employed grounded theory, hinting at coding and categorising activity or reflexive analysis of the field notes without any tangible evidence of how this was done. Choosing and defining the analytical method is central to the initial planning phase. It is closely linked with decisions regarding methodology and method. Analysis exists at a number of different levels, and strategies to sort and manage the collected data form only the most superficial aspect of the process. The final critical stages involve the interpretation of data and its translation into working theories. A range of more structured activities will be needed to bring order to and help identify key issues in the data. On this basis, more creative engagements with the data can take place.

Qualitative research often cannot be easily tidied up. Indeed, I would argue that it should retain aspects of its messy features. Whatever the method of data management, there will always be problems capturing less tangible elements of the interview or observation experience. The process of transcribing interviews can result in the loss of intonation and nonverbal gestures, all potentially expressive of meaning. It can be difficult to convey irony, sarcasm, uncertainty or humour in textual form. Decisions will have to be made about whether and how to capture elements of interaction such as turn taking as well as the construction of the dialogue. Which parts of an observation will be recorded? Would this be done synchronous with the activity, or recorded later but inevitably more selectively? As has been emphasised throughout this chapter, decisions will be determined by the choice of methodology and method. According to these, a study may involve analysis of action, discourse, conversation or narrative.

This chapter does not deal in detail with the mechanics of data management, which are covered comprehensively in most textbooks (Patton, 1987; Punch, 1998). The aim here is to reflect on how to ensure that methods fit the methodology. It is worth emphasising that choices concerning the management of data will need to be made at every stage, from initial data collection to the analysis and writing-up stage. For instance, you need to decide whether your analysis will take place throughout the study to permit emergent themes to inform the content and direction of subsequent interviews, or whether it will be delayed until the completion of the data collection phase.

FINAL REFLECTIONS

Starting out on research involves a series of difficult and challenging choices. You can make the decision trail more coherent and easy to follow by first defining the research question. This in turn will help to define the methodology and method. However, some issues need a great deal of thought and reflection. You will have to probe your own preconceptions, as honestly and openly as possible. You will need to consider why you have come to hold these beliefs. What is it that you want to know? How might this change your opinion? You need to be sure that you have devised a research method that will allow for the unexpected and for evidence that runs counter to your existing opinions.

You also need to look closely at what is motivating you to undertake the study. What are the implications of using other people's time and knowledge to advance your own career or understanding? How might you, or a patient, be compromised by research undertaken during treatment? What are the implications of asking patients to disclose information that you would not normally elicit as part of their therapy? Can you ever be certain that your research will be both ethical and fair? These ethical questions will be examined in the next chapter.

Research choices are not easy to make, but once made they must be explained and justified to the reader. You may find that you made some poor choices or that certain decisions had unexpected or adverse consequences. Again, all these events have to be identified and explained. However, if the research sets out to examine the real, lived world of the participants, it equally exists in a real and lived world of doing research. The choices, the consequent decisions based on events in the study and new directions of enquiry are as desirable as they are often inevitable. You should attempt to take your reader on the journey with you, explaining at every stage how events occurred and how dialogues developed, how relationships were forged and understandings shared. If you can describe and justify what you did, readers have a chance to follow your train of thought and consider whether they would have come to the same conclusions.

REFERENCES

Bogdan, R.C. and Biklen, S.K. (1998) *Qualitative Research for Education: An Introduction to the Theory and Methods*, 3rd edn, Boston: Allyn and Brown.

Crabtree, B.F. and Miller, W.L. (1992) *Doing Qualitative Research: Research Methods for Primary Care*, London: Sage Publications.

Department of Health (2003) 'Research governance', accessed online at www.doh.gov.uk/research/rd3/nhsrandd/researchgovernance.htm, 30 April 2003.

Finlay, L. and Gough, B. (2003) *Reflexivity: A Practical Guide for Researchers in Health and Social Sciences*, Oxford: Blackwell Science.

Law, M., Stewart, D., Letts, L., Pollock, N., Bosch, J. and Westmorland, M. (1998) *Guidelines for Critical Review Forms: Qualitative Studies*. Hamilton,

Ontario: McMaster University Occupational Therapy Evidence-based Practice Research Group.

Lincoln, Y.S. and Guba, E.G. (1985) *Naturalistic Enquiry*, Newbury Park, CA: Sage Publications.

Miles, M.B. and Huberman, A.M. (1994) *Qualitative Research Analysis*, 2nd edn, Thousand Oaks, CA: Sage Publications.

Morse, J.M. (2003) 'A review committee's guide for evaluating qualitative proposals', *Qualitative Health Research*, 13(6): 833–51.

NHS Centre for Reviews and Dissemination (2001) 'Undertaking systematic reviews of research effectiveness: CRD's guidance for those carrying out or commissioning reviews', CRD Report No. 4, 2nd edn, University of York: NHS CRD.

Oakley, A. (1981) 'Interviewing women: A contradiction in terms', in Roberts, H. (ed.), *Doing Feminist Research*, London: Routledge.

Patton, M.Q. (1987) *How to Use Qualitative Methods in Evaluation*, London: Sage Publications.

Punch, K. (1998) *Introduction to Social Research: Quantitative and Qualitative Approaches*, London: Sage Publications.

Seale, C. (ed.) (1998) *Researching Society and Culture*, London: Sage Publications.

Silverman, D. (1993) *Interpreting Qualitative Data: Methods of Analysing Talk, Text and Interaction*, London: Sage Publications.

Sim, J. and Wright, C. (2000) *Research in Health Care: Concepts, Designs and Methods*, Cheltenham: Nelson Thomes.

Steward, B. (2004) 'Writing a literature review', *British Journal of Occupational Therapy*, 67(11): 495–500.

4

Ethical and Governance Issues in Qualitative Research

CLAIRE BALLINGER AND ROSE WILES

Research within any paradigm that includes human participants will inevitably involve choices about how best to satisfy moral obligations to participants while meeting study requirements. Qualitative research raises particular challenges, perhaps because an explicit recognition of the position of the researcher and the research process is fundamental within investigations of this nature. The case scenarios of **Marianne** and **José**, on the next page, illustrate a broad range of issues, including access, informed consent and the inclusion of vulnerable participants.

The aim of this chapter is to focus on the choices to be made around ethical practice in qualitative research, within the emerging context for health research as specified in the Research Governance Framework (Department of Health, 2001). The identification of formal set procedures in ethics applications can mean that the researcher fails to continue addressing the ethical issues on an ongoing basis as the research proceeds (Small, 2001). Small stresses the importance of developing individuals' capacity to make ongoing ethical decisions about the design and conduct of their research. Within this chapter we highlight some of the difficult choices encountered in deciding on best ethical practice, with the aim of encouraging qualitative researchers to think critically about ethical issues relating to their research.

We begin by exploring the scope and boundaries of ethics within research. We then go on to chart the evolution of guidelines for ethical research behaviour, including a brief review of the Research Gover-

Qualitative Research for Allied Health Professionals: Challenging Choices. Edited by Linda Finlay and Claire Ballinger.   Copyright 2006 by John Wiley & Sons Ltd.   ISBN 0-470-01963-8.

Box 4.1 Case studies

Marianne is a psychology graduate employed as a health service researcher on a funded research project. The research aims to investigate how social inclusion of people with learning difficulties is addressed within statutory health care provision and involves multiple research methods. Marianne's particular brief is to gain the views of people with learning disability about their experiences of health care, through a grounded theory approach using interviews.

José is a senior physiotherapist working in a general hospital who is currently studying part-time for a Masters degree and is about to start the project that will form the basis of his research dissertation. José is interested in the culture of the day hospital to which many of the patients with stroke he has treated are referred. He is especially interested in how discharge of patients with stroke from the day hospital is managed. He hopes to explore this through using an ethnographic approach and observing daily nursing meetings, weekly review meetings with the multidisciplinary team and individual intervention sessions with therapists, nurses and doctors.

---

nance Framework in the UK. We next focus in more detail on specific issues likely to be encountered by the qualitative health researcher, and indicate potential solutions to some of these challenges. Throughout this chapter we will use examples from therapy research, and will make reference to the choices and challenges facing Marianne and José (see Box 4.1) as they embark on their projects.

WHOSE ETHICS? WHOSE RESEARCH? THE EVOLUTION OF CURRENT ETHICS PRACTICE

Gregory (2003, p. 2) describes the ethics of research as 'embrac[ing] moral issues rising out of the conduct of research' and proposes the interchangeable use of 'ethical' and 'moral' in relation to research. One has only to consider issues such as homosexuality or the debate around the recent reclassification of cannabis in the UK from a Class B to a

Class C drug to appreciate that what is considered 'morally acceptable' is highly dependent on cultural and historical factors. Similarly, what passes for 'ethical' research practice is highly contingent on the historical climate within which the research is carried out.

If Marianne had been interviewing people with learning disability just a few decades ago, she would have been working with a client group routinely described as 'subnormal' or 'mentally handicapped'. They would have been much less socially visible, typically living in large institutions and generally ignored by the outside world. Social inclusion would have been an alien concept, and it is unlikely that research about issues affecting learning disabled people would have been seen as a priority for research funding. Similarly, the concerns that José is hoping to address through his research have only recently emerged as legitimate and useful topics of research.

Concern with ethical research practice was first widely manifest following the crimes perpetrated by Nazi doctors on people in concentration camps during the Second World War. Evidence of ethical malpractice was also evident in early social research focusing on social processes such as obedience and group norms, Milgram's experiments being some of the most notorious (Milgram, 1963). Determined that such widespread abuse conducted as 'medical research' should end, the World Medical Association drafted the Declaration of Helsinki in 1964 (subsequently revised; see World Medical Association, 2002). The current version of this declaration is founded on the principle that, while health research is recognised as being in the public good, the interests and wellbeing of research participants should remain paramount in any decision about conduct of the research (Montgomery, 2003).

Within the UK, there is no single legal and ethical framework underpinning research practice, although the Research Governance Framework (Department of Health, 2001) has attempted to bring together various guidelines and statutes to provide a coherent context for health research. One of the mainstays of this system continues to be the local research ethics committees (LRECs), established in 1968. Comprising voluntary groups of people with broad expertise and experience, including laypersons, ministers of religion, researchers, clinicians and lawyers, these committees were set up to review medical research proposals in order to determine if they met the criteria for ethical research practice (Peat *et al.*, 2002). The committees' remit included issues such as informed consent, confidentiality and anonymity, risks to research participants and the legal liability of the researcher.

Many of the health professions' own bodies have also developed codes of conduct that include research ethics for the guidance and regulation of their members (e.g. General Medical Council, 2002). As the allied health professions have become increasingly involved in research, they too have either developed their own codes of research ethics or incorporated research ethics into their general codes of conduct (e.g. College of Occupational Therapists, 2003). This has been paralleled by the development of codes of practice for research by organisations representing academic disciplines (British Sociological Association, 2002; British Psychological Society, 2000; Social Research Association, 2003).

The inclusion of professions other than doctors and disciplines other than medicine in the health research arena has introduced a plurality of research paradigms, methodologies and methods. In addition to broadening the topics deemed worthy of research interest, and introducing a variety of ways of conceptualising the research endeavour and the respective roles of the researcher and participant, this plurality has also created tensions around what is deemed acceptable research conduct. Cartwright and Seale (1990), for example, argued that it was inappropriate for ethics committees to oversee surveys of people identified from public records. As they saw it, the fact that their funding body, the Medical Research Council, insisted that they seek ethics approval from their local research ethics committee (which in turn argued that a doctor's consent be obtained before a patient was invited to participate in the research study) reinforced a paternalistic relationship between the doctor and patients, which ran contrary to individuals' civil rights.

RISK AND REGULATION: RESEARCH GOVERNANCE

As a response to inquiries into a series of medical research scandals (Bristol Royal Infirmary Inquiry, 2001; Royal Liverpool Children's Inquiry, 2001) and in an attempt to introduce a more standardised system, the UK government introduced the NHS Research Governance Framework (Department of Health, 2001). This addresses all research carried out by, or involving, NHS staff or NHS resources, and also that carried out by other organisations within health and social care systems.

Research governance within the UK is built around six core principles (Montgomery, 2003, p. 348):

- The rights and safety of research participants must be paramount in any research.
- Independent scrutiny of research plans must occur.
- Participants should be fully cognisant of risks before agreeing to participate – the principle of informed consent.
- Information about participants should be treated confidentially.
- As far as possible, participants should be involved in the design of research.
- Risk should be kept to a minimum.

Under research governance, these principles are enacted through the identification of various protagonists with different responsibilities, namely the principal investigator, the research sponsor, employers, care providers and study participants. The principal investigator has the primary responsibility to the research participants, ensuring that their rights are upheld, that the research team acts according to specified guidelines and that information about participants is kept confidential. The research sponsor is accountable for the quality and management of the research project. Research ethics committees are now a fundamental part of the Research Governance Framework. Their role is also advisory rather than statutory, but NHS bodies cannot permit research to go ahead within their organisations unless projects have received formal approval from a local research ethics committee.

In the next section we highlight some of the choices that qualitative researchers will need to consider in respect to ethical and moral conduct within their project. We have both submitted to and adjudicated on various ethics committees and are aware of the extent to which research governance and LRECs in particular can shape the research venture. We therefore provide examples from our own experiences, and highlight some of the decisions required of the two researchers identified at the beginning of the chapter, Marianne and José. The focus is on four key areas: access to participants, vulnerable participants, informed consent and predicting outcomes of research.

ACCESS TO PARTICIPANTS

Traditionally, the clinical principle that medical professionals have direct responsibility for patients under their care has also extended into the research arena. In practice this has meant that consultants or GPs have exercised control over whether or not their patients may be approached about participation in research projects. However, a number of challenges have disrupted this arrangement, among them the critique of the medical model; greater patient and carer autonomy; and a questioning by the allied health professions of their apparently subordinate position to the medical profession.

Additionally, from a methodological perspective, qualitative researchers are likely to be interested in social processes, which may include investigation of dynamics within the health care team, decision making or patient/client participation. Seeking permission from the medical practitioner before approaching potential participants could have a direct impact on the very focus of study.

In practice these challenges have been interpreted in different ways. Researchers should be aware of the need to negotiate access by including a robust rationale in the information they provide about the study. No clinical setting is under any obligation to provide access, should the demands of the study appear to conflict with best clinical practice. It is courteous to discuss the study with gatekeepers, which may also facilitate the research process through learning about procedures and policies that could influence recruitment, for example. The Data Protection Act (1996) states that the researcher should not know the identity of individuals until they have expressed an initial interest in participating in the study. This usually means that someone present within the setting must initially forward information about the project on behalf of the researcher, thus adding to their workload. Ethically, it is problematic to invite participation from those too ill or confused to take up this offer. Again, this is usually addressed by asking another health professional who knows the patients/clients well to use the inclusion and exclusion criteria by screening out those unable to participate, again adding to their workload. There are therefore many reasons why the researcher might want to talk with key people at the research site prior to starting recruitment.

VULNERABLE PARTICIPANTS

Another key ethical consideration involves decisions regarding procedures to be used with groups of participants who have particular needs or who may be viewed as vulnerable. Ethics committees have a particular brief to protect the interests of such groups. However, while current ethics procedures regard the attribution of vulnerability as

Box 4.2

José, although a novice researcher, recognises potential problems with recruiting colleagues and patients within the setting where he is known. He considers the options open to him. Carrying out the research within another day hospital would be prohibitive in terms of time. However, he feels that it is unacceptable to involve patients whom he has personally treated, even if many of them, he senses, would probably be willing to be asked.

In discussion with his supervisor, he decides to include as the potential focus for his observation only those patients with stroke who have been treated by other physiotherapists. The initial invitation to patients will be made by a day hospital volunteer, who is happy to forward José's written information about the project to those patients identified by the administrator, who is aware of José's entry criteria for recruitment. After discussion with the day hospital manager, José has also requested that he be permitted to give a presentation about his project for the staff at the monthly ward meeting. He will emphasise that no one is under any obligation to participate and that all data will be anonymised and kept securely, away from any identifying information about participants. He also gives an undertaking that he will safeguard anonymity by changing key identifying features in both the research dissertation and subsequent dissemination activities.

unproblematic, classifications such as these might lie at the very heart of the research endeavour.

As an occupational therapist with a background of service provision to people with learning disabilities, I (CB) have based much of my applied work with this group of people on the principle of normalisation (Wolfensberger, 1972). Here, the undesirable position of disadvantaged groups is assumed to have arisen as a consequence of 'socially devaluing' processes and procedures used ordinarily within everyday services. Remedial action would focus on making use of socially valued ways to conduct everyday life (for example in terms of transport usage, communication, leisure activities), typically methods used by the wider general population. However, within the current ethics framework, people with learning disabilities are considered vulnerable. As a consequence there is an expectation that ways of enacting certain aspects of the research project that differ from the 'norm' should occur, focusing, for example, on provision of information about a project or seeking informed consent.

While accepting that such research participants may have special needs, we argue that there should not be an automatic attribution of vulnerability, as such a designation reinforces long-held stereotypes about learning disabled people. The support of an advocate is also not an automatic guarantee that an individual's rights will be upheld and could be viewed as a token gesture included to appease an LREC. The important principle here is that the researcher recognises the complexities of explaining research to potential participants and is committed to expending the necessary time and effort to ensure that individuals understand what is being requested of them, what this may involve and their right to refuse. It is also critical that the individual's modes for communicating assent or dissent are understood.

The requirement for different procedures for disadvantaged groups could not only be ineffectual, but also run contrary to the theoretical position of the individual carrying out the research. The perceived 'vulnerability' or status of learning disabled people as a group could conceivably be the focus of a qualitative research project, being 'sensitive to the social context in which data are produced' (Mason, 2002, p. 3), and might well be actively contested by some of the research participants. Similar issues have been identified in relation to research with children (Alderson, 1995).

INFORMED CONSENT

The principle of informed consent is central to research governance within the UK, and more broadly to the Declaration of Helsinki, the statement that provides the underpinning international framework for research conduct.

The process of enabling informed consent is defined by the Social Research Association as 'a procedure for ensuring that research participants understand what is being done to them, the limits to their participation and awareness of any potential risks they incur' (Social Research Association, 2003, p. 28).

Technically, this refers to consent to participating in the project being fully cognisant of the risks, and also of anything else that might possibly influence the individual's decision to become involved in the research both at the present time and in the future. However, it has been noted that informed consent is understood differently by different disciplines and professions (Alderson and Goodsey, 1998). The requirement for informed consent to participate in research requires the provision of written information about the project together with written consent. Advice from ethics committees about what should be included in participant information sheets has become increasingly specific (see COREC, 2001).

As Montgomery (2003) points out, the rules regarding consent in research have not yet been tested out in law within the UK. While other law exists covering nonconsensual physical contact by researchers, such as administration of a new drug without fully informing a patient/research participant of all possible side effects, the law in respect of qualitative data generation methods is far less clear. Although the principle of informed consent is relatively easy to comprehend, in practice it is not always entirely clear before the study gets under way from whom the consent should be sought. This is notably the case for ethnographies and observational studies set in contexts that see large numbers of different people passing through or where situations are subject to change. Although the governance framework is clear that retrospective consent is not acceptable, it is likely that in some situations it is not possible to identify beforehand who will be participating in the observed action within an ethnographic study.

Several years ago, I (CB) carried out a small empirical piece of research based on ethnographic principles within an NHS day hospital for older people. The ethics form and protocol submitted for consideration by the LREC included an information sheet containing details about the study, written for both staff and patients at the day hospital. Consent to access the day hospital was negotiated with the nurse manager, and fully discussed with the staff at one of their weekly staff meetings. The submission was approved, subject to minor amendments including written permission from the medical director. As several consultant physicians worked with patients within the day hospital, it was unclear to whom this referred, but was discussed and arranged with one of the most frequently visiting consultants.

My original intention was personally to hand all potential participants an information sheet, and give them the opportunity to ask questions prior to the start of the study. However, as there was a fairly rapid throughput of patients and different patients appeared on different days, it soon became clear that this strategy was not practical. I therefore opted to leave the information sheets in the day room for patients to take, and ensured that I was present on multiple occasions so that potential participants were able to talk more with me if they had any queries. At the end of the observation period, I elected to carry out semi-structured interviews with selected participants, and having addressed this aspect within the initial ethics submission, gained full written consent from participants beforehand. This example illustrates how the provision of information, and the opportunity to discuss a study prior to providing consent, may be particularly challenging within some qualitative designs.

Although the situation did not arise, it would have been extremely problematic if any one of the potential participants had not given consent for the observational phase. Should one individual's dissent mean that the entire observational study be abandoned? Or should it mean that only the actions of that particular individual be 'written out' of the fieldnotes? If the latter, what if their activity became a central part of the action that I was observing, such that their exclusion would render the description meaningless? Similarly, José is assuming that if individual members of staff decline to participate, he will be able to exclude reference to them within his observational fieldnotes and elect not to be present to observe during treatment sessions with that staff member. However, this will be problematic if he or she has a key role in the discharge process for an individual participant who has agreed to take part in José's study, for example a key worker who has strong

---

Box 4.3

Within a previous study, Marianne had difficulties with one learn-ing disabled participant in clarifying her role as a researcher as distinct from a 'best friend', which led to personal difficulties for her, particularly as the study ended. Although she thought hard about these issues at the time of the study and worked under supervision, she wonders whether she worked in a manner con-sistent with the principle of informed consent. With more experi-ence, Marianne is now keen to highlight such risks by clarifying her role with potential participants when providing them with information about the study. However, this will be complex, as she is wary of implying that her participants won't understand poten-tially different roles such as 'friend' and 'researcher'.

views about the timing of discharge, or the care package that should be available to support the patient/participant.

PREDICTING OUTCOMES OF RESEARCH

It is considered ethical practice to share with potential participants the expected findings and possible outcomes of a research project, to enable them to assess the benefits of participation. Yet another choice facing the qualitative researcher is how to represent this. As it may be difficult to foresee some of the potential outcomes of qualitative research because of the evolutionary nature of research design within this paradigm, it can be difficult to communicate the potential implications of participating.

One of the potential solutions to this dilemma is to encourage consideration of ethical issues in a process-driven sense, which continues throughout the project (Ramcharan and Cutcliffe, 2001). This might involve seeking a mandate from participants at several different points during the project. José, for example, is conscious that people who have

---

Box 4.4

José has now carried out some fieldwork and is reflecting on his preliminary findings. The LREC agreed that José could include participants with stroke who had cognitive difficulties, providing written consent was also obtained from another representative, such as their spouse or advocate, and evidence was obtained beforehand that they would understand and not be disturbed or distressed by his presence as an observer during any treatments. José's ethics submission stated that he would first consult with the potential participants' key worker to ascertain that they were not likely to become upset, for example because they were emotionally labile. He also decided that the Mini-Mental State Examination (Folstein, Folstein and McHugh, 1975) would be used to ascertain presence of cognitive problems, and that he would exclude those people with cognitive difficulties who were unlikely to understand what was being asked of them, interpreted as a score of 23 or less.

experienced stroke face many daily challenges. These might, in turn, have an impact on their mood, and subsequently influence their decision to participate in his study, or lead to distress or confusion that affects their capacity to retain an understanding of what he is doing. He therefore undertakes to check that participants are happy for him to collect data on every occasion, and also that people are clear about why he is present and what he is doing.

Lawton (2001), who conducted a participant observation study within an inpatient hospice, found that her research design meant that it was not possible to give participants accurate information about a study's focus because it changed during the process of data collection and analysis. Gregory (2003) also notes that the findings of a qualitative research project might look different to those envisaged by the researcher at the start of the project. He argues that, to remain true to the spirit of participant involvement and consent, participants should be consulted about any changing emphasis in the research. In some research approaches this may involve getting interviewees to check transcripts, sharing analysis of data with them and getting their views about conclusions and material to be published (Gregory, 2003).

From a theoretical perspective, the close involvement of research participants accords well with some qualitative research approaches, such as participatory research or action research. However, it is more problematic within other qualitative approaches such as conversation analysis, in which transcription and analysis are carried out in a very detailed way, unfamiliar to many except researchers skilled in this method. A conversation analytic transcription might well be incomprehensible to the participants. We again argue that coherence within a specified research approach or methodology, with inclusion of pertinent references, constitutes an important ethical consideration within qualitative designs.

It might also be possible to encourage researchers to identify the key ethical principles pertaining to their research, and to include examples about how these principles are upheld throughout the duration of the project as a requirement for LREC submissions. Another example suggested by Gregory (2003) is the encouragement of, or provision for, continual dialogue between the principal investigator and research fellow or assistant who may be carrying out the data generation.

In conclusion, this chapter has explored a number of issues raised for qualitative researchers within the current ethics framework and environment within the UK, namely access to participants, the notion of vulnerable participants, informed consent and predicting outcomes of research. Many of the subsequent contributions in this book also allude to ethical challenges within qualitative research, whether through a desire to remain true to own values (see Chapter 13), questioning assumptions about research being exploitative (see Chapter 5) or practical concerns around data collection methods (see Chapter 8). Evidence suggests that many of these issues are also familiar to international qualitative researchers (Cheek, in press).

We have tried to highlight the complex and contingent nature of many decisions regarding ethical research behaviour, and want again to emphasise that the proposed 'solutions' in this chapter are rarely as neat, straightforward or final as the case studies suggest. However, we hope that in the process of exploring the current ethical challenges inherent within qualitative research, we have provided some useful suggestions about how these might be addressed.

REFERENCES

Alderson, P. (1995) *Listening to Children: Children, Ethics and Social Research.* Ilford: Barnardos.

Alderson, P. and Goodey, C. (1998) 'Theories of consent', *British Medical Journal*, 317: 1313–15.

Bristol Royal Infirmary Inquiry (2001) 'The inquiry into the management of care of children receiving complex heart surgery at the Bristol Royal Infirmary', accessed online at http://www.bristol-inquiry.org.uk, 9 April 2004.

British Psychological Society (2000) 'Code of conduct, ethical principles and guidelines', accessed online at http://www.bps.org.uk/documents/Code.pdf, 9 April 2004.

British Sociological Association (2002) 'Statement of ethical practice', accessed online at http://www.britsoci.org.uk/about/ethic.htm, 9 April 2004.

Cartwright, A. and Seale, C. (1990) *The Natural History of a Survey: An Account of the Methodological Issues Encountered in a Study of Life before Death*, London: King Edward's Hospital Fund for London, cited in Bowling, A. (2002) *Research Methods in Health*, 2nd edn, Buckingham: Open University Press.

Central Organisation for Research Ethics Committees (2001) 'Guidelines for researchers, patient information sheet and consent form', accessed online at http://www.corec.org.uk, 24 January 2005.

Cheek, J. (in press) 'The practice and politics of funded qualitative research', in Denzin, N. and Lincoln, Y. (eds), *The Handbook of Qualitative Research*, 3rd edn, Thousand Oaks, CA: Sage Publications.

College of Occupational Therapists (2003) 'Research ethics guidelines', London: College of Occupational Therapists.

Department of Health (2001) 'Research governance framework for England', London: Department of Health.

Folstein, M.F., Folstein, S.E. and McHugh, P.R. (1975) ' "Mini-Mental State": A practical method for grading the cognitive state of patients for the clinician', *Journal of Psychiatric Research*, 12: 189–98.

General Medical Council (2002) 'Research: The role and responsibilities of doctors', accessed online at http://www.gmc–uk.org/standards/research.htm, 9 April 2004.

Gregory, I. (2003) *Ethics in Research*, London: Continuum.

Lawton, J. (2001) 'Gaining and maintaining consent: Ethical concerns raised in a study of dying patients', *Qualitative Health Research*, 11: 69–73.

Mason, J. (2002) *Qualitative Researching*, 2nd edn, London: Sage Publications.

Milgram, S. (1963) 'Behavioral study of obedience', *Journal of Abnormal and Social Psychology*, 67: 371–8.

Montgomery, J. (2003) *Health Care Law*, 2nd edn, Oxford: Oxford University Press.

Peat, J., Mellis, C., Williams, K. and Xuan, W. (2002) *Health Science Research: A Handbook of Quantitative Methods*, London: Sage Publications.

Ramcharan, P. and Cutcliffe, J. (2001) 'Judging the ethics of qualitative research: Considering the "ethics as process" model', *Health and Social Care in the Community*, 9(6): 358–66.

Royal Liverpool Children's Inquiry (2001) 'The Report of the Royal Liverpool Children's Inquiry', available online at http://www.ricinquiry.org.uk/.

Small, R. (2001) 'Codes are not enough: What philosophy can contribute to the ethics of educational research', *Journal of Philosophy of Education*, 35(3): 387–406.

Social Research Association (2003) 'Ethical guidelines', accessed online at http://www.the-sra.org.uk/ethics03.pdf, 9 April 2004.

Wolfensberger, W. (1972) *The Principle of Normalisation in Human Services*, Toronto: National Institute on Mental Retardation.

World Medical Association (2002) 'Declaration of Helsinki', accessed online at http://www.wma.net/e/ethicsunit/helsinki.htm, 9 April 2004.

PART II

Doing the Research

This middle part of the book focuses on different methodologies in action. In 11 separate chapters, various therapy researchers offer their accounts of what it is like to use different qualitative research approaches. In inviting these contributions, our aim was not to provide you, the reader, with models of 'how to do' grounded theory, conversation analysis or whatever. Instead, we hoped these chapters would give you a feel for different methodologies and for the concerns, positions and commitments implicit within them.

We have invited the authors to follow the same structure. Each chapter begins with a section on methodology, followed by ones on doing the research, findings and reflections. We have also encouraged each contributor to explain, and reflect on, their reasons for choosing their particular methodologies. As each author engages reflexively with the challenges involved in doing qualitative research, they highlight different dimensions of the process.

In **Chapter 5**, Mandy Stanley describes a grounded theory study she undertook that explored wellbeing in older people. Mandy's careful description of her method and use of innovative strategies to develop her analysis are noteworthy. **Chapter 6**, written by Barbara Richardson, provides a clear example of how ethnographic methodology can shed light on the characteristics of a culture. Here, everyday practice in physiotherapy is candidly revealed. In **Chapter 7**, Barbara Steward explores some of the dilemmas – and opportunities – created when qualitative and quantitative approaches are combined within a single study. She provides a spirited defence of this distinct choice. In an elegant account of her use of conversation analysis, Ruth Parry in **Chapter 8** convincingly introduces us to a methodology as yet little used within AHP research: conversation analysis. She identifies its use in improving interactional practices within therapy as a potential benefit. Michael Curtin, in **Chapter 9**, provides an honest and thoughtful description of the challenges he faced when using a biographical approach with children. He considers some exciting alternative ways of re-presenting his research findings. In **Chapter 10**, Sarah Dean, together with Sheila Payne and Jonathan Smith, provide insights into another relatively new approach within therapy research: interpretative phenomenological analysis (IPA). The authors' careful working of the different stages of analysis helps capture the systematic and layered nature of interpretation within this methodology. A different but similarly layered approach to interpretation is developed in **Chapter 11** with reference to a wider group of colleagues and research allies. Here, the biographic-narrative-interpretive method is skilfully represented by Tanya Campbell-Breen, with Fiona Poland. Anne Killett's commitment to empowering the young people who have contact with her service is evident through her persuasive use of participatory research, in **Chapter 12**. Privileging an ethical relationship in this way is not without its challenges, a point she makes well. The potential for artistry and poetry within qualitative research is highlighted in **Chapter 13**, where Linda Finlay shows how existential phenomenology deepened her understanding of her participant's experience of a chronic deteriorating condition. Claire Ballinger and Julianne Cheek, in **Chapter 14**, provide an exciting example of how postmodern research approaches, in this case discourse analysis, can unsettle the familiar by challenging conventional ways of making sense of shared notions such as risk. Paula Hyde's contribution, in **Chapter 15**, explores another intriguing but under-utilised research approach. Her informal checking of meaning with various players in the research process provides a thought-provoking example of how psychodynamic interpretation is co-constituted within qualitative research.

We encourage you to dip into the various chapters in this part as a way of becoming familiar with the different approaches described. It is likely that you will feel affinity with some of the authors while finding the arguments of others less persuasive. We would urge you, however, to see your response as a product of your own epistemological preferences. Such reflection – far removed from making value judgements about a particular author's research – will, we hope, help you shape your future research endeavours.

5

A Grounded Theory of the Wellbeing of Older People

MANDY STANLEY

'You've got to have faith.' This was my mantra while I was conducting my study for a PhD and grappling with how to actually do a grounded theory study. I read and reread the classic texts but still struggled, particularly with how to do the analysis. I was not looking for a recipe but some examples of how to actually 'do' it. In this chapter, I hope to offer other researchers such an example. I will draw on my own use of grounded theory in a study to explore older people's perceptions and understandings of wellbeing to help readers comprehend the use of grounded theory in research practice. I have included descriptions and examples (such as the interview questions I used and how I analysed my data) in the hope that, besides being useful to others, these will add to the available literature on grounded theory. To conclude the chapter I will discuss the ethics of using in-depth interviewing as a data collection approach with participants who might be perceived as vulnerable.

METHODOLOGY

Roberts and Taylor (1998, p. 102) define grounded theory as an approach that 'starts from the ground and works up in an inductive fashion, to make sense of what people say about their experiences, and then to convert those statements into theoretical propositions'. For

Qualitative Research for Allied Health Professionals: Challenging Choices. Edited by Linda Finlay and Claire Ballinger. Copyright 2006 by John Wiley & Sons Ltd. ISBN 0-470-01963-8.

example, grounded theory has been used to study the process of death and dying in hospitals (Glaser and Strauss, 1965), women with post-partum depression (Beck, 1993) and people with bipolar depression (Hutchinson, 1993b). The aim of grounded theory is to generate a mid-range theory that is 'grounded' empirically, that is grounded in the data collected. The approach was developed by two sociologists, Barney Glaser and Anselm Strauss, in the 1960s.

There are different inflections to grounded theory, many of them deriving from developments of the original Glaser and Strauss concept. In later years the two sociologists differed over developments in the approach to grounded theory, to the point where Strauss developed a version of grounded theory with Corbin (Strauss and Corbin, 1990). This was criticised by Glaser, who argued that it no longer constituted grounded theory (Glaser, 1992). However, others disagreed with this view. (For a more detailed examination of the differences between Glaser's approach to grounded theory and that of Strauss and Corbin, see Annells, 1996.) Other variations have been described by Stern (1980), Charmaz (1994) and Eaves (2001), among others.

The therapist researcher who wants to use grounded theory needs to be aware of the nuances of different approaches and take a considered and argued position with respect to the inflection used. For my study I chose to use what is known as the traditional Glaser and Strauss approach (Glaser and Strauss, 1967). This is essentially the same as the later Glaserian position (Glaser, 1992). I chose this because I had discovered myself to be quite a 'purist'.

THEORETICAL ORIENTATION

Grounded theory is informed by symbolic interactionism. Many sociologists, philosophers and psychologists have influenced the development of symbolic interactionism, most notably George Herbert Mead and Herbert Blumer. Bowers (1988, p. 36) has defined symbolic interactionism as 'a social-psychological theory of social action'. It focuses on the individual as a socially constructed being, and on the processes of social interaction by which individuals make sense of the world.

Drawing on the tenets of symbolic interactionism, grounded theory assumes that people order and make sense of their world, even when it appears to be disordered. Reality is therefore a social construct. In grounded theory the researcher looks for processes that are going on in social situations and studies these in order to arrive at a theory that explains the action in the social context under study (Stern, 1980).

Grounded theory is particularly useful in areas where little is known about the phenomenon of interest or where there are few existing theories to explain an individual's or group's behaviour.

When I began my PhD study I reviewed the relevant occupational therapy and gerontological literature (Stanley and Cheek, 2003). It was evident that older people's views of what constitutes wellbeing had not been studied, that the literature contained few references to it, and that current representations of wellbeing in the literature were lacking in empirical support. It was also evident that occupational therapists and those with an interest in the field of gerontology did not have a clear, widely accepted view of what wellbeing is for older people. This appeared incongruous given that wellbeing is a central concept to the occupational therapy profession (Reed and Sanderson, 1999). My study therefore aimed to address the gap in the literature and to generate a theory about wellbeing based on the views of older people themselves.

The lack of congruence in the literature about a definition of wellbeing suggests that it is a complex concept. Some of the complexities derive from the fact that individuals vary considerably in terms of personality, life situation and the society in which they live. Grounded theory provides a way of exploring the inter-relatedness of all these conditions.

DOING THE RESEARCH

Grounded theory questions focus on process. As such, they are often 'how?' questions: for example, how do occupational therapists go about their work? How do occupational therapists define and use evidence? They may also be 'what?' questions. In my study, for example, the central research question was: 'What are older people's perceptions and understandings of wellbeing?'

DATA COLLECTION

While various methods and techniques are used to collect data in grounded theory, these often involve in-depth interviews or participant observation, or a combination of both. I chose to use in-depth interviews in my study as it was not feasible to observe older people to gain insight into their perception of wellbeing. I sought an exemplar to guide my question development, as I needed to make sure that my interview questions fitted with the grounded theory focus on process and social actors. It is difficult to find examples of the questions that grounded theory researchers actually use in their interviews, but I found those used by Hutchinson (1993b) and I modelled my questions on these, as follows:

1. In order to understand you a bit better, tell me about how you spend your day.
2. As you know, I am interested in finding out about the perceptions and understanding of wellbeing of older people. So if I said to you 'What does wellbeing mean to you?' what would you say?
3. Tell me, how do you achieve wellbeing?
4. What difficulties do you encounter in achieving/maintaining wellbeing?
5. What advice would you give to a person who is not experiencing wellbeing?
6. What would you like to tell health care professionals about wellbeing for older people?
7. What would you like to tell your family and friends about wellbeing?
8. What would you like to tell politicians and governments that would improve the lives of older people?
9. Is there anything else you would like to comment on about wellbeing?

In addition, basic demographic data was collected about respondents' age, gender, living situation and suburb.

I conducted semi-structured in-depth interviews with 15 participants who were all 75 years or older and living in the community. Participants included both males and females and were recruited through opportunistic and snowball sampling. They varied in terms of their living situation, socioeconomic status and marital status. However, the aim of sampling was to explore and extend the theoretical constructs of the emergent theory rather than to obtain a representative sample. Interviews were conducted in the participant's home.

ANALYSIS

In grounded theory, as soon as data collection begins, so too does analysis. While analysis of data is presented here in a linear fashion, illustrated with examples from my study to demonstrate how I got from the transcripts to a core category and basic social process, it bears emphasis that doing grounded theory is much more of an iterative process.

Data collection and analysis occur simultaneously. The researcher then returns to the field, in my case to do more interviews and collect more data for analysis.

I chose a traditional Glaserian approach to analysis. While Strauss and Corbin (1990) probably provide a more structured approach for the novice grounded theorist, the more traditional Glaserian approach is more closely aligned with the theoretical orientation of symbolic interactionism. I wanted to remain consistent with the theoretical orientation, as it seemed to fit with my views of how knowledge is constructed.

Constant Comparative Analysis

Data analysis begins with the researcher analysing a transcript or field-notes line by line and assigning '*in vivo*' codes. An *in vivo* code is a word or a short phrase that describes what is happening, often quite close to the original words of the participant. It can range from the simple and concrete to the complex and abstract. For example, the line of transcript 'I think just to, to enjoy your life within your capacity. And everyone has limitations on their capacity haven't they, and limitations on their interest too' (Joan) was coded 'enjoy life within your capacity'. Put simply, coding is the process of sorting, labelling and organising the data (Charmaz, 1994).

In the case of my own research, large numbers of codes were generated in this way. By the time I had coded the first three interviews I had over 45 codes. I re-examined each of these, recoding some and subsuming others into another code. For example, 'being positive' and 'positive outlook' became one code, 'being positive'.

Data collected in a grounded theory study is analysed using constant comparative analysis (Glaser and Strauss, 1967). This involves coding a unit of data and comparing it with all the other units of data coded in that category. It is a systematic tool for developing and refining the theoretical properties of a category, and if applied rigorously will assist the researcher to move from a simple description of the participants' categories to a theoretical level (Seale, 1999).

As further interviews were conducted and transcripts produced, I continued with the open coding. These transcripts were either coded using the existing codes or, if new data emerged, a new code was created. As the data collection and analysis progressed the codes were compared with each other and organised into clusters according to fit. These clusters were then labelled as categories. For example, 'staying in own home' and 'value independence' became the category 'maintaining independence'.

Selective Coding

Following open coding I moved to selective coding. This involves a much more conscious search for the core category, and is at a higher or more abstract level of coding. Use of constant comparative analysis continues, enabling the researcher to compare the emerging categories, and collapse them into more abstract categories (Stern, 1980). For example, in my study I grouped the emerging categories of 'financial security', 'feeling safe and secure' and 'being comfortable' under a single category label of 'being comfortable and secure'. The codes 'importance of family', 'importance of friends' and 'belonging to a club' were combined into the category 'being connected'. In the early stages of analysis it may be difficult to understand how the codes are connected to each other. This is often a cause for much consternation: as a researcher I can remember doubting that I could ever draw the loose ends into a coherent theory. Gradually, however, through a process of thinking, consulting and talking, coherence does begin to emerge.

Theoretical Coding

The next step in analysis is theoretical coding. Glaser (1978) suggests that theoretical coding is used to reveal the conceptual relationships between categories. To assist with analysis, I began to draw diagrams in order to try to reveal some of the relationships between the categories. Discussing the diagrams with peers, along with continued use of the constant comparative method, enabled me to further refine and clarify the relationships between categories and begin to identify the core category. It also enabled me to see where I needed to do further theoretical sampling. Glaser argues for the use of theoretical coding families to assist the researcher to see relationships among categories. One of these coding families is the 'six Cs': the examination of categories in terms of their causes, consequences, contexts, contingencies, covariance and conditions.

Theoretical Sampling

Theoretical sampling is employed as data gathered in the early stages of research are analysed and emergent themes arise (Glaser and Strauss, 1967; Glaser, 1992). The categories in the emerging theory determine where and from whom the next data are to be collected. Informants are sought who are thought able to contribute further data relating to the important emerging theoretical constructs so that these can be examined and elaborated further. Glaser and Strauss (1967, p. 47) suggest that 'the basic question in theoretical sampling is: What groups or subgroups does one turn to next in data collection? And for what theoretical purpose?'. Those questions guide the researcher as to which cases to study, which people to interview or which settings to observe in order to find things that might challenge and/or extend the emerging theory (Seale, 1999). Different questions may be asked of different participants as the theory evolves. Grounded theorists also theoretically sample the literature at this stage.

Memoing

In grounded theory, memoing is seen as a way of preserving emerging ideas and hypotheses about the data as analysis is conducted. As ideas strike the researcher they are recorded in the form of a memo. If ideas are not recorded at the time they may well be forgotten and lost. Bowers (1988, p. 51) states, 'Memoing is a crucial process for the grounded theory researcher'. Memos are used to raise the data to a level of conceptualisation (Grbich, 1999) and to locate the emerging theory within existing relevant theoretical frameworks (Glaser, 1978). Memos themselves are also sorted and further memos written as the theory is developed (Grbich, 1999).

During the analysis stage of my study I wrote memos in order to be consistent with the grounded theory approach. An example of a memo I wrote early in the analysis process reads as follows:

8th October
Routine
Each of the people interviewed so far, when asked to describe how they spend their time give a description of the routine. They usually start with what time they get up and dressed for the day and also include the time they usually go to bed at night. There is variety in the amount of routine that is described. Some have routine in the day, others it is more commitments on different days of the week, or month. Connects to Ferol Ludwig's study of how routine facilitates wellbeing for older women. Leads to the question about how much variety in an individual's routine leads to wellbeing? Can a highly routinised person, that is one who follows exactly the same routine every day, experience wellbeing? Can a person who doesn't appear to have any routine in their life experience wellbeing?

Writing the memos engages the researcher in a process of reflexivity. Reflexivity is defined by DePoy and Gitlin (1998, p. 230) as 'the process of self examination' and by Mason (2002, p. 5) as 'thinking critically about what you are doing and why, confronting and often challenging your own assumptions, and recognizing the extent to which your thoughts, actions and decisions shape how you research and what you see.' The researcher examines his or her own perspective and determines how this has influenced what has been learnt in the study and how it is learnt. The purpose of reflexivity is not to establish neutrality but to achieve a far more intense insight.

FINDINGS

CORE CATEGORY

Grounded theorists search for the social processes present in human interactions (Hutchinson, 1993a). The researcher is trying to identify a core category: one that arises from the data, to link the various pieces of data together, and one that explains much of the variation between data (Hutchinson, 1993a). Discovery of a core category is a requirement for a quality grounded theory study (Hutchinson, 1993a). The core category is somewhat like a central theme and becomes the basis for the generation of theory. A core category is linked to as many other categories as possible, occurs frequently in the data, takes longer than any other category to achieve 'saturation' (the point at which no further data emerge) and has explanatory power for the total analysis (Glaser, 1978). While all grounded theory studies will have a core category, not all will reveal a basic social process. The basic social process is similar to a core category, except it has two stages or phases that account for process or change over time (Glaser, 1978).

In my own study, as my theory of wellbeing began to emerge I could see that some categories appeared to have reached 'saturation': in other words, no further data were emerging. I had had a hunch for some time that 'perceived control' might be the core category and I was aware that the core category was usually the last to achieve saturation. I therefore set about interviewing further to test my idea out. I sought participants who might be in situations that would challenge their ability to maintain perceived control. These might be people who had health challenges, were at risk of losing their independence or had experienced a significant loss such as the death of a spouse. During the analysis I kept coming across expressions of actions that seemed to me to be examples of 'tradeoff': situations where participants gave up something but replaced it with something else. I began to suspect that tradeoff was a basic social process.

However, I was hesitant to declare it as such. I was expecting to find a core category, but I was not necessarily expecting to identify a basic social process. Only a few of the grounded theory studies that I had read had been able to define a basic social process. I turned to the literature to look for examples (see for example Rose, Mallinson and Walton-Moss, 2002; Wilson and Morse, 1991). After finding some, I went back through each of my transcripts and made notes on how the participants had used tradeoff. I also generated further interview questions to probe the finer details of the process. For example, while I knew that participants used tradeoff, did it come from their perceiving that they were in control? Or did tradeoff itself create the perception that they were in control? At this point I went back through each transcript and generated a chart that identified how each participant used tradeoff, what had caused this and with what consequences. In grounded theory, the basic social process is expressed in the form of a gerund. As Fagerhaugh (1986, p. 135) points out, 'Gerunds suggest movement and change, or process over time.' Having established 'tradeoff' as a basic social process, I therefore changed its name to 'trading off'.

A diagrammatic representation of the relationships between the core category 'perceived control', the other categories and the basic social process 'trading off' is presented in Figure 5.1. Analysis of the data revealed the categories 'personal resources', 'feeling comfortable and secure', and 'it is up to me' as providing a basis for older people to face the 'challenges to equilibrium', and for them to use the basic social process 'trading off' to achieve 'perceived control', and thus wellbeing.

A 'challenge to equilibrium', such as a health problem or loss of a relationship, threatens the participants' ability to perceive that they are in control. The challenge prompts older people to review their 'personal resources'. The category 'personal resources' consists of the properties 'having good health and good fortune' and 'being engaged and active'. Personal resources can be used to buffer the challenges to equilibrium. Older people also need to feel 'comfortable and secure' in their immediate environment and local community as part of their perception of being in control. Part of adjusting to a change in circumstances or loss of capacities involves taking the attitude 'it's up to me'. Older people with such an attitude are able to appraise their choices, engaging in 'trading off' to achieve perceived control and thus wellbeing.

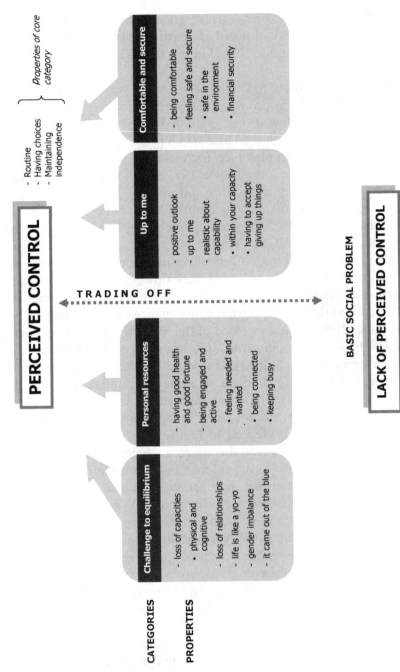

Figure 5.1 Diagram of core category and relationships between categories

THEORETICAL SATURATION AND SAMPLE SIZE

It is not possible to predict the sample size prior to commencing a grounded theory study. Data are collected until no new codes or categories emerge, thus achieving what is termed saturation. By achieving saturation the researcher ensures that the theory accurately reflects the situation and the result is a rich, 'thick' description. When I came to the fifteenth interview in my study I began to feel quite sure that I was not hearing anything that would dissuade me away from what I had defined as the core category. While I collected further data within each of the categories, nothing new emerged. This fifteenth interview made me feel confident that I had reached saturation for all the categories and could therefore stop interviewing participants.

DATA MANAGEMENT

Effective management of large amounts of textual data generated by my study was a constant challenge. Once data gathering began, I had to make a decision about how I was going to manage not only the data collected but also the analysis, including the recording of an audit trail. I investigated the use of computer software, but decided that the benefits of using a commercially available means were outweighed by the disadvantages of cost and the learning time required to master the program. I had also read cautionary tales against over-emphasising codes and categories and thereby generating variable analyses, which were removed from the situational context. Such an approach would be more aligned with a positivist theoretical orientation and therefore not appropriate for my grounded theory study. Richards and Richards (1998) note that it is important not to let software determine the form and content of the interpretive activity. As my own preferred learning style is very visual and 'hands on', I probably made the right decision to tackle analysis manually, even if there were frequent occasions on which I regretted this decision.

Later in the analysis, when conducting further interviews, I cut a copy of the transcript into pieces. I then placed the new statements from the transcript against the previous codes. At this stage, too, I drew diagrams or 'mud maps' of the codes and the relationships between them (see Figure 5.2). (A 'mud map' is an Australian expression for a rough-drawn diagram that is not to scale.) In this context, my mud maps were somewhat like concept maps. Another form of mud map was kept on the wall of my work office and stimulated conversation about the

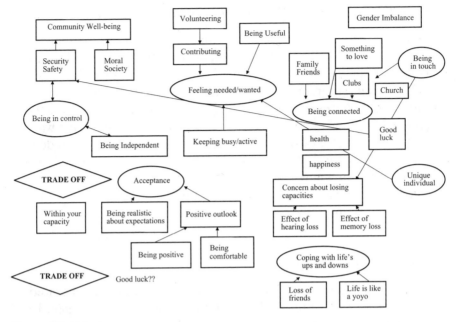

Figure 5.2   Mud map

analysis with my colleagues and students. The conversations assisted me in clarifying the codes and categories and the relationships between them. Numerous diagrams were drawn as data were repeatedly compared. As a result, a number of codes were collapsed into categories and renamed. The diagrams also enabled me to explore the relationships between categories in the search for the core category. These diagrams, too, formed part of the audit trail: a strategy for ensuring credibility and trustworthiness.

REFLECTIONS

CRITIQUES OF GROUNDED THEORY

Postmodernists criticise grounded theory for its affinity with positivism (Grbich, 1999). They argue that coding, the first step of analysis in grounded theory, de-contextualises the data and forces the researcher to adopt a 'narrow' view of the data. According to Seale (1999, p. 103), postmodernists 'equate grounded theorizing with an attempt to impose a single, exclusive interpretation of data', rather than acknowledge that there may be multiple realities. However, such a critique could equally be levelled at other qualitative interpretive methodologies. The debate is as much about philosophy as it is about grounded theory.

Grbich argues that in the health area researchers have used grounded theory to generate theory 'that is little more than an affirmation of their own biases' (1999, p. 180). However, I would argue that this criticism is as much about 'sloppy method' or 'method slurring' as about grounded theory. Good grounded theory is not about imposing pre-existing theories, it's about generating theory that is grounded in the data. To avoid 'method slurring', researchers are advised to make explicit which version of grounded theory they are using and to describe – and justify – any deviation they make from the chosen approach (Cutcliffe, 2000). Stanley and Wise (1990) argue that it is not possible to generate theory that is entirely grounded in the data as all researchers come to the research study with experiences, ideas and values – all of which influence the analysis and thus the theory generated. Obviously researchers are not 'clean slates'. In grounded theory analysis they must use processes to ensure that the theory really does emerge from the data and is not forced. Conversely, Glaser (1992) suggests that it is the researchers' professional and personal experience together with their in-depth knowledge of the data that gives them the sensitivity to generate categories. Keeping detailed audit trails and making the analysis process transparent at the writing-up stage strengthen the position of the grounded theory researcher.

ETHICAL ISSUES

Ethical approval for my study was sought and gained from the Human Research Ethics Committee, University of South Australia. The study was conducted observing all the usual ethical procedures of informed consent, observation of confidentiality and anonymity and the protection of the rights of participants. During my reading and thinking about the use of in-depth interviews I came across two specific ethical issues that had relevance for my study. The first issue related to my interviewing people who could be perceived to be vulnerable. The second one, closely related to the first, was the ethics of inviting myself into people's lives and expecting them to divulge personal information without having an ongoing relationship with them and without their getting any direct benefit from participating in my study.

Russell (1999, p. 403) has addressed the issue of interviewing vulnerable older people by posing the question: 'Should we be "mining the minds" of these disempowered people for our own research purposes?' She suggests that it might be more ethical to offer more than a 'hit and run intrusion'. In my own case, I was very mindful of the power I had as a researcher. However I would argue that the people in my study were not particularly vulnerable or disempowered. They were all living independently in the community and were free to exert their own free will about whether or not to participate in the study. They also had the freedom to choose how much they divulged in their responses to the interview questions. I would argue that if we continue to see older people as vulnerable then we are reinforcing negative societal perceptions and expectations (Russell, 1999).

As a researcher I was aware of the responsibility to be sensitive to the power that I potentially held as 'the interviewer from the university'. It is not possible to equalise the power relationship between the researcher and those being researched, but the differential may be reduced by close scrutiny of what is being studied, why it is being studied and who is to benefit from the research (Suto, 2001). Carpenter and Whalley Hammell (2001) suggest that the resultant knowledge needs to be placed at the disposal of the researched as well as the researchers. Mindful of this, I produced a summary of the key findings, in accessible language, and made this available to all participants. One participant received a complete copy of the thesis at her own request.

As to the issue of the older person not benefiting from involvement in the study and the researcher being the main person to benefit from the relationship, in common with Russell (1999) and Kvale (1996) the participants in my study found the interview to be an enriching experience and were reluctant to end each session. The participants appeared to enjoy telling their story and to have the opportunity to reflect on their life experience.

CONCLUDING REFLECTIONS

One of Glaser's catch cries is 'trust in emergence'. At many points in my analysis I would remind myself of this and tell myself I just had to have faith that it would happen. What I have attempted to do in this chapter is to reassure the reader that, with perseverance, thinking, writing and talking, the theory will 'emerge' from the data. It will coalesce into a set of theoretical propositions that have 'grab' and 'fit'; that is, they will make sense to those reading them and appear to fit the real world.

In this study, grounded theory was used to explore, in all their complexity, the perceptions and understandings of wellbeing held by a group of older Australians living in the community. The resultant mid-range theory has implications both for occupational science knowledge and for occupational therapy theory and practice. These will be published elsewhere. Grounded theory, in my view, enables therapist researchers to derive a theory specific to therapy practice that is properly grounded in the lives of participants.

REFERENCES

Annells, M. (1996) 'Grounded theory method: Philosophical perspectives, paradigm of inquiry, and postmodernism', *Qualitative Health Research*, 6(3): 379–93.

Beck, C.T. (1993) 'Teetering on the edge: A substantive theory of postpartum depression', *Nursing Research*, 42(1): 42–8.

Bowers, B.J. (1988) 'Grounded theory', in Sarter, B. (ed.), *Paths to Knowledge: Innovative Research Methods for Nursing*, New York: National League for Nursing.

Carpenter, C. and Whalley Hammell, K. (2001) 'Evaluating qualitative research', in Whalley Hammell, K., Carpenter, C. and Dyck, I. (eds), *Using Qualitative Research: A Practical Introduction for Occupational and Physical Therapists*, Edinburgh: Churchill Livingstone.

Charmaz, K. (1994) 'The grounded theory method: An explication and interpretation', in Glaser, B.G. (ed.), *More Grounded Theory Methodology: A Reader*, Mill Valley, CA: Sociology Press.

Cutcliffe, J. (2000) 'Methodological issues in grounded theory', *Journal of Advanced Nursing*, 31(6): 1476–84.

DePoy, E. and Gitlin, L.N. (1998) *Introduction to Research: Understanding and Applying Multiple Strategies*, 2nd edn, St Louis, MO: Mosby.

Eaves, Y.D. (2001) 'A synthesis technique for grounded theory data analysis', *Journal of Advanced Nursing*, 35(5): 654–63.

Fagerhaugh, S. (1986) 'Analyzing data for basic social processes', in Chenitz, W.C. and Swanson, J. (eds), *From Practice to Grounded Theory: Qualitative Research in Nursing*, Menlo Park, CA: Addison-Wesley.

Glaser, B. (1978) *Theoretical Sensitivity*, Mill Valley, CA: Sociology Press.

Glaser, B.G. (1992) *Basics of Grounded Theory Analysis: Emergence vs Forcing*, Mill Valley, CA: Sociology Press.

Glaser, B.G. and Strauss, A.L. (1965) *Awareness of Dying*, London: Weidenfeld and Nicolson.

Glaser, B.G. and Strauss, A.L. (1967) *The Discovery of Grounded Theory*, New York: Aldine de Gruyter.

Grbich, C. (1999) *Qualitative Research in Health: An Introduction*, Sydney: Allen & Unwin.

Hutchinson, S. (1993a) 'Grounded theory: The method', in Munhall, P.L. and Oiler Boyd, C. (eds), *Nursing Research: A Qualitative Perspective*, New York: National League for Nursing Press.

Hutchinson, S. (1993b) 'People with bipolar disorders' quest for equanimity: Doing grounded theory', in Munhall, P.L. and Oiler Boyd, C. (eds), *Nursing Research: A Qualitative Perspective*, New York: National League for Nursing Press.

Kvale, S. (1996) *Interviews: An Introduction to Qualitative Research Interviewing*, Thousand Oaks, CA: Sage Publications.

Mason, J. (2002) *Qualitative Researching*, 2nd edn, London: Sage Publications.

Reed, K.L. and Sanderson, S.N. (eds) (1999) *Concepts of Occupational Therapy*, 4th edn, Philadelphia, PA: Lippincott Williams & Wilkins.

Richards, T.J. and Richards, L. (1998) 'Using computers in qualitative research', in Denzin, N.K. and Lincoln, Y.S. (eds), *Collecting and Interpreting Qualitative Materials*, Thousand Oaks, CA: Sage Publications.

Roberts, K. and Taylor, B. (1998) *Nursing Research Processes: An Australian Perspective*, Melbourne: Nelson.

Rose, L., Mallinson, R.K. and Walton-Moss, B. (2002) 'A grounded theory of families responding to mental illness', *Western Journal of Nursing Research*, 24(5): 516–36.

Russell, C. (1999) 'Interviewing vulnerable old people: Ethical and methodological implications of imagining our subjects', *Journal of Aging Studies*, 13(4): 403–17.

Seale, C. (1999) *The Quality of Qualitative Research*, London: Sage Publications.

Stanley, L. and Wise, S. (1990) 'Method, methodology and epistemology in feminist research processes', in Stanley, L. (ed.), *Feminist Praxis: Research, Theory and Epistemology in Feminist Research*, London: Routledge.

Stanley, M. and Cheek, J. (2003) 'Well-being and older people: A review of the literature', *Canadian Journal of Occupational Therapy*, 70(1): 51–9.

Stern, P.N. (1980) 'Grounded theory methodology: Its uses and processes', *IMAGE: Journal of Nursing Scholarship*, 12(1): 20–3.

Strauss, A. and Corbin, J. (1990) *Basics of Qualitative Research*, Newbury Park, CA: Sage Publications.

Suto, M. (2001) 'Issues related to data collection', in Whalley Hammell, K., Carpenter, C. and Dyck, I. (eds), *Using Qualitative Research: A Practical Introduction for Occupational and Physical Therapists*, Edinburgh: Churchill Livingstone.

Wilson, S. and Morse, J.M. (1991) 'Living with a wife undergoing chemotherapy', *IMAGE: Journal of Nursing Scholarship*, 23(2): 78–84.

6

An Ethnography of Physiotherapy Culture

BARBARA RICHARDSON

The undergraduate education programme plays an important role in the professional socialisation of students in preparation for practice, but more information is needed on how students build on their learning when they start work as juniors. As a physiotherapy educator I wanted to enquire into the process of applying knowledge to practice in workplace settings. I wanted to explore features of practice that may influence and crucially shape practice development. In any group of people the behaviour, patterns and beliefs that constitute standards for deciding what is, what can be, how one feels about it, what to do about it and how to go about it constitute the culture of that group (Goodenough, 1971, cited in Patton, 1990). I wanted to explore the culture of physiotherapy.

In order to identify and illustrate how interactions between practitioners can shape physiotherapy practice, I needed a research approach that would allow me to find out how people behave in social groups in natural practice settings. Ethnographic methodology was appropriate because it aims to promote an understanding of why people behave as they do and it combines naturalistic models of enquiry with an interpretive approach to analysis of data, making it possible to reveal culture as shared knowledge and as acquired social behaviour (Wolcott, 1999; Hammersley and Atkinson, 1995).

My study of physiotherapy practice, carried out a number of years ago, comprised three components: a questionnaire survey of the

Qualitative Research for Allied Health Professionals: Challenging Choices. Edited by Linda Finlay and Claire Ballinger. Copyright 2006 by John Wiley & Sons Ltd. ISBN 0-470-01963-8.

understanding that qualifying students have of their profession; a study of reflective diary extracts and interviews with three newly qualified juniors in their first year of practice; and a study of the clinical practice of three senior physiotherapists. Together these provided an ethnographic account of the role of the workplace environment and of social interactions in practice development. This chapter will focus on the third of the three components. I will explain how taking an ethnographic approach to the study provided a suitable theoretical base for looking closely at practice activities and the inter-relationship of people in groups. I will discuss how the study can be evaluated for the knowledge it adds to an understanding of the professional development of junior physiotherapists in workplace cultures of practice.

METHODOLOGY

Taking an ethnographic approach to design of my study was in line with the ontological view (Brewer, 2000) that people's actions are based on their personal and individual perceptions and interpretation of events around them at any one time, and from this basis of shared behaviour the culture of a group of people emerges (Savage, 2000). Work organisations are a meeting place of groups of people in a complex, fluid world of social interaction. The continual change in interactions from one minute to another shapes the way people think and the way they behave.

Relating theory to my study, I assumed that the physiotherapists constructed the reality of their world and that their interpretation of their experiences with others governed their behaviour. From my experience as a practitioner and from discussions with students, I saw that the ways senior physiotherapists work, including their rationale of practice and their behaviour, were central to understanding the culture of physiotherapy practice. Following the tenets of naturalistic qualitative inquiry I purposively (Pope and Mays, 2000) selected routes of investigation to gain the information I saw as important to describe physiotherapy practice. I chose to study three clinical areas of work: with older people, with outpatients and work in the community. I considered these to be rapidly developing areas in which changes in health care would be important to the future practice of physiotherapy. I selected one practitioner in each area who had been qualified for more than three years, by which time I thought their views and understanding of their practice would be well established. I identified people with whom I had some acquaintance over a period of time, believing this would facilitate a good working relationship.

Observation in the field, the fundamental method of ethnographic studies, was essential to my study. It was only from first hand experience of 'being there' that I could explore the dynamics of social interactions as they took place (Brewer, 2000). I wanted to provide a rich, inclusive account of how workplace activities and practitioners' views weave together. Observational methods of data collection gave me an in-depth understanding of some of the complex phenomena in health care interactions within a particular workplace context. I was able to access the fine detail of work activities (Brewer, 2000), and this enabled me to see how the physiotherapists actually organised their time and how they behaved (despite what they might say). I could note non-verbal behaviours, who talked to whom, at what times and for how long. I observed the therapists' use of language at certain times with certain groups and I saw how they organised and adorned the physical workspace of their rooms and offices.

The other mainstay of data collection in ethnography is interviews. Through these, I could further explore the thinking and reasoning of individuals with a view to more closely portraying and interpreting the behaviour I noted in the observations. In-depth interviews helped to capture detail of the physiotherapists' perspectives and experience. My interest was not in whether or how many times they carried out certain activities, but rather in investigating what they said and why and how they said it (Giacomini and Cook, 2000). Their personal, spontaneous responses provided valuable insights into their thinking and enhanced my observations of how they carried out their professional role, their processes of clinical decision making and the professional stance they took. Their responses also provided insights into the symbolism implied by their workload organisation (Pope and Mays, 2000). Taken together, these created discernible patterns of behaviour and relationships within this social group of physiotherapists. I looked at how these individuals interacted in their specific area of practice. I followed them when they were working by themselves and when they were in social interaction with others. I then placed what I had learnt about their work within a wider perspective: that of its possible significance for the culture and wider profession of physiotherapy.

There were several important choices to make in preparation for the study. Defining the focus of the study and the research question was the first, because it guided the initial choice of participants and the way I made decisions at any number of stages during the research. I also had to choose which activities and treatment sessions to observe or to ignore.

A fundamental principle of ethnographic research is to work closely with people to try to understand their behaviour (Pope and Mays, 2000). The trustworthiness of my data collection and the veracity of the information I gleaned depended on the rapport I established with my participants. I needed to gain their confidence, while they needed to be reassured of the credibility and legitimacy of the study to which they were contributing. The challenge was to explain clearly my position in the research so that they would not only feel able to relax and act normally during the research process, but also feel sufficiently confident to disclose their opinions and beliefs (Smith, 1996a). The credibility of the research (including how my role in it was perceived) was critical during the early stage of gaining access to the research site and to the participants.

Negotiation with the prime gatekeepers (Pope and Mays, 2000) – in this case the clinical managers – and gaining the approval of local ethics and research governance committees are important ethical processes. Approval for accessing the research site depended on the assurances of confidentiality and anonymity that I gave for both person and location throughout the study and in any future publications relating to it. My negotiations with the participants were based on the decisions that I anticipated I would want to take at various stages of the study. I might want to extend an observation period to include other areas of interest, such as a staff meeting or an in-service education session. I might need to do this so as to focus on one or two specific behaviours: perhaps the process of taking patient histories, or the process of working with other professionals. These types of decisions, I knew, would shape the emerging design of the research. I therefore recorded them in a reflective diary, knowing that this would help me identify a decision trail at a later stage. This would add to the rigour of any report I wrote on the study and it could also assist the analysis of my own impact on the research as an observer (Smith, 1996a).

Field analysis techniques require investigators to consider explicitly how their own presence might influence findings (Giacomini and Cook, 2000). I needed to account for any research bias in my analysis and presentation of findings that might be inferred by my relationship with the participants. While I could not remove the potential for my presence to influence proceedings, I could in the way I set up the study actively try to minimise it. I chose to meet the participants a number of times in order to discuss the research process and map out a plan for the observations. I explained the aims of the data collection and how I would behave during the various stages of the study.

There are no standardised descriptions of qualitative studies because each one is unique, varying according to the people involved, the specific research focus and the events that occur. I was particularly conscious that I would be taking into the project my understanding of physiotherapy, as well as my knowledge of the participants. This could provide the basis of a trusting relationship, one that should allow me access to high-quality data. This relationship would, I hoped, enable me to identify and present details of practice that would strike a resonance with other practitioners in other workplaces. However, it could also influence the way I represented the data and thus act as a potential source of bias.

As Patton (1990) points out, it is useful to consider variations in observation in terms of a continuum. At one end of this is the full participant observer, an insider who is completely immersed in the situation and who intimately shares the life and experiences of the group. At the other end is the nonparticipant observer, essentially an outsider and onlooker. I chose an intermediate position on the continuum, adopting a collaborative approach in which I took the role of a participant observer who was an educator and researcher exploring the participants' perceptions of students' learning needs. I hoped this would give me opportunity to gain an in-depth and comprehensive view of their activities as experts without making them feel judged. Keeping a reflexive account of my interactions as a researcher was important. Besides acting as a continual source of introspection, the reflexive diary would help me guard against making premature assumptions about what was happening (Mays, 1995): assumptions based on my own views of physiotherapy.

DOING THE RESEARCH

In carrying out my research, I was mindful of my ethical responsibilities. The need for a basic description of practice in which to ground theory had to be set against the danger of encroaching on the sensitive territory of patient/professional interaction and interactions between the multidisciplinary team. The development of a protocol for 'practitioner observations' and a data release form for patients who agreed to take part in the study assured the confidentiality and anonymity of their data. These steps also recognised the unpredictability of health care interactions and the need to establish protocols for practitioners that would enable them to understand their right at any time to veto observations or take any action they felt necessary to protect the patient or themselves as professionals.

To collect my data, I negotiated a research design that included several full-day observations over a period of weeks. I wanted the schedule to include cycles of treatment intervention in which I could observe assessment, treatment and progression of treatments. It was agreed that I would use various methods to record events, dialogue or descriptions of the setting, including observation, interviews and video recording.

My observations focused on events that I thought would help me understand the practitioners' frames of reference in a specific setting of physiotherapy practice: for example their routine activities, or activities that were identified as unplanned. I recorded the length of time given to taking a case history alongside the time given to teaching home exercises or other forms of education. I also recorded snatches of dialogue, noting the language used at particular stages of giving advice and the tone of voice (e.g. whether personal or authoritarian). I was mindful, too, that important information can be gleaned from noting events and behaviours that might be expected but that do not actually occur. I was conscious that the degree of sensitivity I achieved in my observations would be my most valued resource and my best tool for gathering insights (Schatzman and Strauss, 1973). I also recognised that my educational interests would direct my data collection. Aware that my study would be one of comparatively few studies of practice, I felt it important to strive to include as many everyday activities as possible. This, I believed, would help reveal the complex underlying structures of people's interactions.

When making observational fieldnotes, I did not follow a procedure set by prepared checklists geared to noting particular timed events, or particular behaviour. Conscious of the wide differences in practice settings, I made general notes related to the specific setting. At this exploratory stage I wanted the data sources to help construct a broad preliminary picture of practice that subsequent research studies could investigate further, perhaps through the observation of specific phenomena.

My fieldnotes were augmented by taped interviews. I would often set these up when the observations prompted questions. Sometimes it was important to understand what was happening without delay. For example, I needed to grasp the application of an unfamiliar respiratory technique so that I could appreciate its use during the day. At such times, I would hold a quick interview in the corridor or by the nursing station between patient visits.

I made video observations of each participant carrying out a patient assessment and a patient treatment. This was done to facilitate a recall that could prompt their reflections on their practice. Video-recall techniques allow a micro-analysis of some of the characteristics of specific practice environments, gestures and body language. They can also provide insight into practitioners' understanding of their own practice by 'making the familiar strange' (Sarangi and Roberts, 1999).

My enquiry process was iterative; that is, I collected data, analysed them to develop tentative theories of what was happening, and then collected further data to clarify my ideas. My conceptual framework of analysis was based on dimensions of the practitioners' paradigms of practice: I looked for features in the data that reflected their thinking about the purpose of their practice, how they carried the work out and the outcomes they expected. Specifically, I looked for the knowledge they perceived to be important to them: the ways they interacted with their patients, the procedures they adopted for diagnosis, the models of practice on which they based their treatment, the ways they delivered their service, the goals and aspirations they had for their clients, and their views on their own professional development needs. The analysis of data started in the field when I began to focus on particular aspects of practice such as the time spent with patients, or participants' understanding of the complexity of tasks. This led me to collect further data that helped to refine my ideas of how the physiotherapists valued and prioritised their work.

When it came to the final analysis stage, I could draw on my field-notes, my reflective research log, interview transcripts and the transcripts of participants' analysis of their own data. The data from these different sources provided the base for a triangulation (Patton, 1990). Through constantly comparing data (Hammersley and Atkinson, 1995) across the sources I was able to ensure that the ultimate interpretation and theory developed from the data and adhered closely to reality. I tried to be continually alert to my biases and to the subjectivity shown in my being drawn to some data and not others. I was constantly on the lookout for omissions and conflicting ideas. It was important to make as transparent as possible the process of abstracting from the raw data. This enabled me to show how themes emerged and how they were grounded in the context of the study, thereby adding to the rigour of the study and the validity of the emerging themes.

Transparency enabled me to show the development of preliminary analytic categories relating to the environmental setting, the activities of a typical day and the views of the participants. On the basis of these categories I was able to identify an exemplar of practice in each area of work, in which the details of the physical environment and the organisation of practice were shown to be relevant to the cultural background of practice. The analysis at this stage was further helped by the participants' own coding of some of their data, relevant to the professional development of juniors. From this analysis I was able to identify certain common themes: attitudes towards professionalism; attitudes to care; and perceptions of professional development.

FINDINGS

The exemplars of practice were three work environments: a care of the elderly ward, where one or two physiotherapists were surrounded by a number of other health care professionals; an outpatients department, where large groups of physiotherapists worked together in isolation from other health care professionals; and an example of community work, where a sole-charge physiotherapist worked largely isolated from other health care professionals. The exemplars highlighted practitioners' perspectives of practice and the small group cultures they developed.

In the case of the care of the elderly work environment, the culture of the physiotherapy department appeared to dominate the physiotherapists' concept of themselves as professionals – despite the fact that they spent comparatively more time as part of a multidisciplinary team. When they emerged from the physiotherapy department, where they met with their colleagues and had their personal lockers, they spoke of going 'out on the wards'. The work was portrayed as following a daily routine that could be disturbed by events on the ward. In-service training sessions promoted the development of physiotherapy skills rather than application of those skills in a social context of care.

In contrast, the culture of practice in the outpatients setting, which was isolated geographically from the rest of the hospital, presented an orderly, structured environment in which the activities of the day could be predicted with confidence and controlled. There was little direct interaction with other health care professionals other than contact by phone with general practitioners. In-service training concentrated on developing physiotherapy techniques. Tutorials for juniors, something not seen in the care of the elderly setting, were given great importance, with periods of time formally blocked off for them each week.

In the community work setting, the culture of practice was that of a single practitioner, isolated from the hospital environment and from other physiotherapists. Here, the practitioner's car – in which considerable time was spent – served as an office as well as a means of transporting equipment from place to place. The practitioner's awareness that she was working in the context of the multidisciplinary team was important to her maintaining contact with necessary personnel, whether social services technicians, GPs or nurses. Workload was seen as variable according to need and each day was carefully planned, thought through and prioritised. Professional development was carried out through reading journals and books and through exchanging views and ideas with a colleague using email.

Attitudes to care showed similar variation. In the outpatients' setting, for example, there was strong opposition to any attempt to reduce the time spent with individual patients despite the pressure to cut waiting lists. The community physiotherapists' examination techniques were described as 'the pits', on the grounds that they made it possible for them to get only 'a few bits of information' and therefore just to guess what was wrong with patients. In the outpatients' setting, technique and skills were seen as paramount in problem solving. It was regarded as important for juniors that they did not have 'a false impression that they come out knowing everything – because it is easy to get caught out'. While they placed value on attending courses, practitioners thought that this should not occur during the first year of practice, when every junior, irrespective of need or ability, was expected to consolidate their learning.

The attitude to care among physiotherapists working on the care of the elderly ward focused on maintaining a daily routine with specific patients while also being ready to respond on a minute-by-minute basis to events on the ward as part of the team. The minutiae perceived necessary for attention on the ward could lead to the unplanned work often severely interrupting the planned work and a priority given to clearing a 'patient load' for the day. The resulting little use of gym activities when patients needed to be taken off the ward was justified on the grounds that time was better spent ensuring that patients on the ward 'had a good walk, an educational walk'. In the community the attitude to care, characterised by an emphasis on patient participation and collaboration, was obvious in the little 'hands-on' work in the 'assessment and advice' service, which was clearly based on patient empowerment.

The view was expressed that 'many physiotherapists enjoy doing things to others and curing somebody but there are few things to cure and rather we [in the community] help people and help nature to cure'. Despite this philosophy, however, the amount of time spent with each patient in the community was judged against the time perceived to be spent with patients in an acute service rather than in terms of the individual's need.

The ethnographic interviews provided evidence of an argument in defence of each approach to practice. This argument referred to an acute care model of practice or to practices demonstrated in initial training, which could have taken place several years earlier. There was a common concern among the physiotherapists to deliver a full service of care to patients within the constraints of their professional time. The amount of time spent with each patient was judged against some pre-conceived idea of what was correct. However, it was not clear whether this judgement was made in relation to the individual patient's need or to some ill-defined norm of acute service delivery against which every-thing was seen to be inadequate. These practitioners also appeared to be in agreement that junior staff were limited in the contribution they could make to clinical practice until they had 'hands-on experience'. They made no differentiation in the complexity of tasks; the profes-sional consensus expressed was simply on the time needed in clinical experience to ensure competence. Their paradigms of practice were dominated by the need for skills-based practice to develop competence. While aware of the move towards evidence-based practice, they did not feel it their own professional responsibility to contribute to this. There was little in the data to show any awareness of a potential need to change their practice.

Ethnographic accounts can be a rich source of insight into the lives of a group of people, but they can only portray life as it is, not how it should be. My role as researcher was to interpret or transform these accounts (Sword, 1999) in relation to my research focus. Taking an ethnographic stance in the collection and analysis of data enabled me to assess the extent to which practitioners' views of physiotherapy prac-tice could potentially influence the development of juniors. My findings suggested that junior staff can be exposed to a range of perspectives on practice and that these can vary according to the specific hospital or practice setting. For example, in one context the task of walking patients might be seen as the domain of the expert, while in another it might be understood as a routine task that could be dealt with by physiotherapy assistants. The fact that assistants were little used in outpatient work in this study may well have contributed to the overall impression that outpatient work was complex and would be a struggle for juniors to cope with. In contrast, the wider use of physiotherapy assistants in community practice may have contributed to an impression that the work there was less demanding and exacting.

My interpretation of these ethnographic accounts raised questions about the nature of experiential knowledge and how it is communicated in developing the practice knowledge of juniors. It also raised questions about the extent to which, in the early years of practice, a balance is struck between the 'indoctrination' of juniors and encouraging them towards autonomous practice. I concluded that at graduation students need strong paradigms of practice against which they can evaluate their development and influences on it.

REFLECTIONS ON RIGOUR AND TRUSTWORTHINESS

My concern throughout the study was to ensure its rigour and trustworthiness. Adopting a largely realist epistemological stance, I wanted to be sure that I captured 'real' practice. However, I couldn't just be an objective, unbiased researcher. I was implicated at every stage of the study, and managing this became my continuing challenge. I wanted my observer notes to become the 'ears, eyes and perceptual senses for the reader' (Patton, 1990, p. 26) to ensure that the data I collected would take a reader of my research into the heart of the working culture of physiotherapists, into the 'way of life' of an identifiable, socially interacting group (Sword, 1999).

Conventionally, ethnography is used in anthropological studies to focus on a group that is notably 'strange' to the observer (Pope and Mays, 2000). My familiarity and intimacy with the group I studied were both problematic and an advantage. The choice of my research status as a participant observer gave me the opportunity to view at close range the behaviour and opinions of 'actors' in the field. It also increased my awareness of current health care issues. It was difficult to maintain a neutral line of questioning in some interviews, where practitioners vehemently opposed approaches to practice that I as an educator embraced. At such times the need to shift from the 'clinical gaze' of the educator to the 'ethnographic lens' of the researcher (Lawlor, 2003) was uppermost in my mind.

The rigour of my analysis rested on recognising that, on the one hand my biases could colour my findings, and on the other awareness of my biases could make me particularly sensitive to nuance and detail. For this reason it was important for me to conduct a continual, reflexive evaluation of the choices I made in the process of analysis and interpretation. I wanted to construct a basic description of practice in which to ground theory relating to a sensitive area: that of patient–professional interactions and of interactions between multidisciplinary team members (Sword, 1999; Brewer, 2000). The development of a protocol for observing practitioners as well as a data release form for patients who agreed to take part in the study not only assured the confidentiality and anonymity of data (Smith, 1996b), it also recognised the unpredictability of health care interactions and the need to establish protocols for practitioners to clarify their right at any time to veto observations or take steps to protect patients or themselves as professionals.

Each observational study – by its very nature unique – poses both ethical challenges and challenges related to deciding on the value of the research (Savage, 2000). Procedures that establish trustworthiness, such as the clarity of the insider/outsider position of the researcher and how that is dealt with, should be taken into account (Sword, 1999). The possibility of a passive observer being a disturbing presence has long been recognised (Schatzman and Strauss, 1973), but the presence of an observing student in health care settings is not unusual. That I was already known to the participants could enhance the trustworthiness of the data collection. Although it was impossible for me to throw off my 'insider' identity as an educator, I requested to be treated simply as a 'fly on the wall' who would not be expected to interact with other practitioners, medical staff or patients unless called on to do so. I wore an appropriate name badge but no physiotherapy uniform. The care I took not to present myself as a challenge to the practitioners' judgements or authority helped strengthen the authenticity of the data collection.

In all observational studies, maintaining a critical distance and avoiding 'going native' can prove problematic (Pope and Mays, 2000). However, my prolonged engagement in the field added to the internal validity of the study and the trustworthiness of the observation data, in that I could be sure I was observing phenomena of importance in that setting. Offering participants choice about their degree of involvement, for instance through member checking to agree on the authenticity of data or for comments on emerging themes, added further validity to the analysis of data (Hammersley and Atkinson, 1995). Ultimately, the external validity of my research rested on my detailed and varied data collection and analysis. I was able not only to strike resonances with other settings but also to provide a decision trail or road map. This, I hoped, could be followed by others in their own workplaces (Giacomini and Cook, 2000) to obtain comparable data relevant to their own settings methods.

In summary, adopting ethnographic methodology provided a relevant theoretical basis for the collection and analysis of data, because it acknowledged situated action at work (Richardson, 1999) and the possibility of identifying key work interactions and patterns of thinking in individual perspectives that can contribute to the corporate culture of physiotherapy practice. This allowed me to take into account the tacit and explicit knowledge shown in everyday social interactions in the workplace and to determine multiple perspectives and influences that can shape a physiotherapy work culture.

Carrying out field observations in an ethnographic study provided a means of describing the culture of physiotherapy practice towards the goal of developing a theory of professional development. In my view, this could not have been achieved or gleaned through personal accounts (narratives) in diaries or interviews alone. The ethos of health care now increasingly recognises the quality issues of interactions among health care professionals, which are contingent on high standards of individual client-focused care. It cannot be denied that our sense of the social world is shaped by the sense of what can be written about it (Atkinson, 1992). Ethnographic qualitative research studies can provide detailed accounts of practice and insights to prompt further scrutiny of practice.

REFERENCES

Atkinson, P. (1992) *Understanding Ethnographic Texts*, Newbury Park, CA: Sage Publications.

Brewer, J.D. (2000) *Ethnography*, Buckingham: Open University Press.

Giacomini, M.K. and Cook, D.J. (2000) 'Users' Guides to the Medical Literature XXIII, Qualitative research in Health Care B: What are the results and how do they help me care for my patients?' *Journal of American Medical Association*, 284(4): 478–82.

Goodenough, W. (1971) *Culture, Language and Society*, Reading MA: Addison-Wesley.

Hammersley, M. and Atkinson, P. (1995) *Ethnography: Principles in Practice*, 2nd edn, London: Routledge.

Lawlor, M.C. (2003) 'Gazing anew: The shift from a clinical gaze to an ethnographic lens', *American Journal of Occupational Therapy*, 57(1): 29–39.

Mays, N. (1995) 'Qualitative research: Rigour and qualitative research', *British Medical Journal*, 311: 109–12.

Patton, M.Q. (1990) *Qualitative Evaluation and Research Methods*, 2nd edn, Newbury Park, CA: Sage Publications.

Pope, C. and Mays, N. (2000) 'Observational methods in health care setting', in Pope, C. and Mays, N. (eds), *Qualitative Research in Health Care*, 2nd edn, London: BMJ Books.

Richardson, B. (1999) 'Professional development 2: Professional knowledge and situated learning in the workplace', *Physiotherapy*, 85(9): 467–74.

Sarangi, S. and Roberts, C. (1999) *Talk, Work and Institutional Order*, New York: Mouton de Gruyter.

Savage, J. (2000) 'Ethnography and health care', *British Medical Journal*, 321: 1400–2.

Schatzman, L. and Strauss, A. (1973) *Field Research: Strategies for Natural Sociology*, Englewood Cliffs, NJ: Prentice Hall.

Smith, S. (1996a) 'Ethnographic enquiry in physiotherapy research 1: Illuminating the working culture of the physiotherapy assistant', *Physiotherapy*, 82(6): 342–9.

Smith, S. (1996b) 'Ethnographic enquiry in physiotherapy research 2: The role of self in qualitative research', *Physiotherapy*, 82(6): 349–52.

Sword, W. (1999) 'Accounting for presence of self: Reflections on doing qualitative research', *Qualitative Health Research*, 9(2): 270–8.

Wolcott, H.F. (1999) *Ethnography as a Way of Seeing*, Walnut Creek, CA: AltaMira Press.

7

Investigating Invisible Groups Using Mixed Methodologies

BARBARA STEWARD

In this chapter I offer an account of the difficulties I experienced in selecting an appropriate methodology for my PhD research. I eventually used both quantitative and qualitative methods, but struggled to work out how to integrate their contradictory findings.

The first problem I confronted was finding out about a group of people, teleworkers, concerning whom little was known. I first encountered teleworkers when I worked as a community occupational therapist and met clients working at a distance from a conventional office. They considered that their work had a negative effect on their health and wellbeing. They had been told that telework would bring positive results, reducing the stress and fatigue associated with commuting while allowing active engagement in convivial family life. In reality, they had found that their 'invisibility' and absence from the workplace led them to feel depressed and isolated.

Teleworking developed in the 1960s, growing as an employment option as computer systems improved and dissatisfaction with commuting increased. It presented a cost-effective option for employers to reduce office costs along with sickness absenteeism. A better work–life balance (Ahrentzen, 1989), more autonomy and flexibility (Comfort, 1997) and improved career opportunities for women (McGrath and Houlihan, 1998) were among its purported benefits. Critics sceptical of such hopes (Pile, 1993) had no hard evidence to support their positions, with the result that opinions ranged from utopian to dystopian views of teleworking as an employment option. Roe (1998, p. xvii) suggests that 'while convenient as a notion into which everyone could project his or her desire, telework appeared to suffer from an evasiveness and lack of substance when it came to research and practical work'. Research, where it existed, was located within business, labour market and employment policy studies and were predominantly quantitative in approach. The voices of teleworkers themselves were inaudible in the debate.

From a pilot study I conducted, it was clear that, unlike other groups brought together by some acknowledged common feature (such as diagnosis, life event or social grouping), many of the participants did not subscribe to a shared definition of themselves as workers. Many did not define themselves as teleworkers and appeared unfamiliar with this term as an employment category. Telework has been defined in the literature as 'remote working' (Probert and Wacjman, 1988), as a new-age cottage industry (Toffler, 1980) and as a way to make 'human beings whole again, working and living in the same community' (Huws, 1984). Where other studies might be located in fields of shared understanding of the medical or social context, this study of telework had no clear foundation. My supervisor observed that I was working at the cutting edge of very muddy waters (Bellaby, 1999)!

The research thus posed a number of methodological problems. The participants were anticipated to be almost endlessly diverse: employed, self-employed or unemployed; working full- or part-time: volunteers or conscripts; in new, transient or long-established telework schemes; at home or elsewhere in remote satellite offices. The demographics of teleworking were hugely contested: while some studies indicated just a few hundred thousand people teleworking in the UK, others placed the figure at several million. Qvortrup (1998, p. 21) suggests that measuring their numbers is like 'measuring an elastic band. The result depends on how far you stretch the definition.'

My pilot study indicated a huge diversity of work experiences and a constant flux of people entering and leaving home-based work. Many participants had teleworked for less than two years, occupying marginal positions within their companies or the labour market. Some described telework as a privilege, which they avoided putting at risk by reporting illness or taking sickness leave. Self-employed and unemployed workers avoided being recognised as homeworkers, which carried a negative business image. As a result, many stated that they felt that they were invisible to their managers, colleagues or customers because they worked at home and/or chose to avoid drawing attention to themselves by asking to take sickness leave.

Conscious of these many complications, I narrowed down the focus of my research by seeking to pursue two questions: What is telework in the eyes of those who say they are doing it? And how are health, illness and sickness defined and experienced by people who are working this way?

METHODOLOGY

MIXING QUANTITATIVE AND QUALITATIVE APPROACHES

As I started my research, I was confronted by a critical problem. My two research questions demanded different methodologies. The first indicated an approach by which events might be quantified and patterns of telework engagement identified. In the absence of evidence or shared understandings about what teleworkers did on a day-to-day basis, I needed to gather information about the context in which to locate and comprehend participants' narratives. I needed to have at least some idea about what teleworking involved. The second question, in contrast, offered opportunities for participants to describe and explain the meaning of the lived experience of telework in their own words and in their own way. I struggled with the conundrum of whether these antagonistic approaches could or should be married (Bryman, 1988; Brannan, 1992). The quantitative element felt at the time like a life raft, providing substance and structure against which to evaluate what teleworkers said they were doing or what their employers were expecting them to be doing. Was it possible to conduct a study from reductionist and critical realist perspectives at the same time?

Various ways have been suggested to combine qualitative and quantitative methodologies. It is often recommended that qualitative research precedes quantitative surveys, to establish the items for the questionnaire. Conversely, statistical results may identify issues that require subsequent examination through in-depth, qualitative interviewing. Some theorists suggest that numerical analysis can be applied to qualitative data through counting the frequency of codes and categories (Loos, 1995). If added up, these are said to provide evidence of the strength and reliability of the emerging themes (Kuiken and Miall, 2001). However, qualitative researchers appear to view switching between them as more controversial and problematic (Fielding and Schreier, 2001).

I was clear that I wanted to explore the 'structural' features of telework organisation as well as the 'processual' aspects of teleworkers' lives (Bryman, 1988). To what extent, I wondered, could these two views be brought together within one research project? Alternatively, would it be possible for me to switch between two methodologies? Normally phenomenological research brings clusters of similar comments or observed incidents together while acknowledging that the same words or concepts mean different things to different people. A frequency approach assumes that the use of a word or phrase indicates a shared meaning, and that the researcher is uniquely placed to assume valid synonymous meanings for elements of the data from which reliable numerical value can be derived. This requires a considerable leap of faith: that identical meanings can be attached to elements of observation or interview data drawn from a number of study participants.

Mixed methodologies are often analytically combined through triangulation, a validation method that compares different types of data from different perspectives or sources to estimate whether these corroborate one another (Seale, 1998). Kelle (2001) suggests that triangulation can achieve either the mutual validation of results or a fuller, complementary picture of the phenomenon. Triangulation assume if data tally, the researcher should be more assured of their veracity. However, Hammersley (1983) emphasises that there is a gulf between confidence and certainty. Do people report the same information using different research methods? Might not enumeration and triangulation encourage a search for convergence that ignores idiosyncratic data? Do matched data carry more weight in a final analysis than contradictory ones?

My expectation was that the two sets of data, one based on quantitative questionnaires and the other on in-depth semi-structured interviewing, would provide complementary evidence to be analysed and presented for participant validation.

DATA COLLECTION AND ANALYSIS

If any valid and reliable quantitative data were to be gathered about telework, decisions would have to be made concerning the size and representative selection of the sample for statistical analyses. Could I find a sample size among these elusive employees and self-employed workers that was adequate to the needs of statistical analysis? How could a representative sample be identified from a group of workers about which so little was known? In the unlikely event that such conditions could be met, would it be possible, or appropriate, to interview that number of subjects through in-depth interviews on their work and health? Would it then be possible to return for a second interview to explore participant validation? It seemed to me that the essential conditions for a statistical analysis could not be met. At the same time, it struck me that each participant gathering their own quantitative data might enrich the investigation.

In due course I decided that my qualitative interviews should establish themes that would be explored further via quantitative questionnaires. I rationalised that teleworkers' work diaries and calculations of time worked and time off sick, although numerical in nature, were in many respects as qualitative as interview data. Data analysis would involve collating the records from quantitative questionnaires, but then using them in a hermeneutic project that would allow each participant to explore and explain their own questionnaire data. Here I was not attempting to find causal relations or test hypotheses. The collection of events and patterns of work would provide one more dimension to help participants explore and define telework with me.

I became increasingly confident that my 'mixed methodologies' would enable participants to examine their own teleworking lives in a number of different but complementary ways. Using multiple types of data and data collection would enrich participants', and my own, exploration of multiple meanings and interpretations. As it turned out, contradictory sets of evidence were generated by individuals using these different approaches, which provided a rich source of evidence through which participants discussed shifting, ambivalent views of their teleworking lives.

Within my university department, there was heated debate about whether I should, or indeed could, undertake inferential statistical analysis on the basis of data from the 40–50 teleworkers I intended to access. My supervisor was keen that if I was collecting quantitative evidence I should demonstrate an understanding of its statistical analysis. There was a fear that examiners might expect this. The departmental statistician was adamant that the numbers were insufficient, and correctly pointed out that I had never intended to apply more than descriptive analysis to individual data. It was tempting to consider producing what would be seen as hard evidence about these workers, especially to a business audience where such telework research results would be welcomed. However, this aim would have driven the research process away from the phenomenological study I wished to undertake.

DOING THE RESEARCH

As the research got under way, a range of difficulties quickly emerged. Invisible workers are hard to identify! I read reports of company telework schemes, only to find that these had been temporary or involved only a few privileged workers whom the companies preferred not to name. Unemployed teleworkers using computers at home for black-market enterprises were clearly keen to remain anonymous. The self-employed often hid the fact that they worked from home because they said that the lack of formal office premises implied a 'Mickey Mouse' company. My definition of telework as 'people using computers to work at home' encouraged some people to volunteer who only worked odd days away from the office, but were keen to present their view of distance working. I decided to set a parameter of 50 per cent of total work hours spent working at home. In practice, however, this proved difficult to apply when working with the participants. Was it 50 per cent of a week, a month or a year? The invisibility of what workers did at home, the lack of clarity about how they organised their lives and the relative novelty of this type of work indicated that I would need to explore changes in their lives and experiences over a prolonged period of time. I wanted to see these people and where they worked. I also needed to negotiate trust in our relationship over time.

The participants proved to be an elusive group. Many were acquired through 'snowballing' (Bogdan and Biklen, 1982), gathering names of teleworkers from people already enrolled onto the study. Often these people did not define themselves as teleworkers at all and needed reassurance that they fitted the criteria. This was despite the fact that they confirmed they worked predominantly at home through the use of a computer. I must admit that my fear of having too few participants, together with my growing awareness of the undefined nature of this form of working, led to increasing latitude in the inclusion criteria. Once recruited, however, participants actively engaged in the project and many described valuing a rare opportunity to discuss their work lives. I was sometimes concerned that an element of support and counselling developed in our relationship because they were isolated and invisible. None of the 44 participants was a patient and all of them knew me only as a researcher. Many, however, were keen to know if they were 'typical' or if their problems were commonly encountered by others.

The first stage of the study took the form of an in-depth interview. This explored the factors that had determined participants' choice of working at home and their views of telework as an employment option. Five questionnaires were then sent to participants at intervals throughout a nine-month period. These aimed to provide a sequence of 'snapshots' of specific elements of their emerging telework life identified from the analysis of the first round of interviews. These elements included hours and days worked, sickness absence, and periods of domestic and leisure activity. They recorded the organisation of time and space, domestic and family events, work–leisure balance, periods of illness and sickness absenteeism. The first interview and the questionnaire data were provisionally analysed and a short report of this analysis was posted back to individuals in preparation for discussion in a follow-up interview. The aim was to move beyond simply checking the authenticity of the data towards exploring new areas and new levels of analysis (Bloor, 1983).

Although only 11 per cent of participants dropped out during the course of the longitudinal project, there were significant shortfalls in participants' responses. Questionnaires were often returned incomplete. In some cases, they did not allow participants to record the type and quantity of their work experiences. Many participants, too, found writing their diary entries time consuming or difficult. These problems in conceptualising the type of work and the way they worked and accurately recording it became important aspects of the discussion in the follow-up interviews. The missing data proved as interesting for us to explore as those entered in the questionnaires.

FINDINGS

Collecting data on the basis of different methods proved especially useful in exploring the content and nature of teleworking life. Participants frequently mentioned that they had never before attempted to record or examine how they worked. They also discussed the impact this was having on them. The recording of 'factual' data, even if this remained a subjective assessment not 'proven' by researcher observation, enabled participants to self-report on their activities and provide data that we could discuss. Apparent contradictions in the questionnaire and interview data offered a hook for discussions, which examined what participants had recorded at the time and how they had subsequently come to construct events.

The completed questionnaires provided valuable data on the nature of teleworking. Much of this could not have been predicted on the basis of the existing literature. The expected implications of being employed or self-employed for wellbeing proved to be less important than the extent to which the participants were absent from a conventional workplace and colleagues and invisible at home to others as 'legitimate' paid workers. The returned diaries showed periods of the day spent making physical contacts with employing companies for formal meetings and social events, followed by extended hours of work at home.

These findings indicated that teleworking affected the construction and boundaries of work time and place. Time boundaries were extended into what would have been commuting time and domestic and leisure time at weekends. Participants reported that this went beyond the extent of flexible working hours they would have undertaken in their previous conventional office lives. The loss of a commute and an external office and fixed or well-defined working hours influenced their own and others' perception of them as workers. As one participant said, 'If you are based at home, people don't see what you are doing. You are just not at work.' Working at home not only rendered them invisible to colleagues, it also cut them off from an everyday office, which no e-communication could replace.

Teleworkers' invisibility and absence from the office environment also raised issues of trust and trustworthiness. They reported feeling that they were perceived by colleagues and employers to be less trusted than conventional employees. Loss of trust between employers and colleagues, or teleworkers and their customers, was widely described. Such lack or diminution of trust appeared to create difficulties for teleworkers when managing illness or taking sickness leave. Unless others witnessed a teleworker's premorbid or post-illness symptoms claims, the worker felt their illness to be unconfirmed by others and their sickness not legitimised. However, being away from others appeared to allow teleworkers greater autonomy and flexibility in managing their symptoms and this permitted work to continue, even if in a modified form during periods of illness. As one participant put it, 'I had a temperature for a day, so I went to bed for an hour and worked the rest. Before I would have been encouraged to take a day off.'

While teleworkers could avoid the risks associated with taking sickness leave, this in turn created a perception of teleworkers as being especially healthy. This limited their opportunities to admit to being ill. One participant told me: 'If I am ill I shouldn't work. That is the employer's view. Whereas if I am here [at home], they think I can work.'

Although they recorded periods of illness and time off work in their diaries, in interviews many participants were adamant that they had not been off sick. Some refused to believe that they had recorded illness or sickness in their questionnaires and had to be shown the entries. When shown these, some expressed shock and still failed to recall recorded incidents. Others explained that they had been unwell but not ill, and had therefore recorded periods of being 'under the weather' but still 'at work'.

A number of possible explanations were considered for the apparent mismatch between questionnaire data and interview discussion. It is possible that participants failed to understand the question and reported all minor illnesses rather than sickness absence from work as requested. It appeared that concepts of illness and sickness were poorly differentiated and although teleworkers slowed their work rate or took part of a day off work, rarely did they take a whole day off sick. Discussions suggested teleworkers were beginning to categorise illness and sickness in different ways to how they had done previously as conventional office workers. The collation of the quantitative evidence proved vital to debate these changing experiences and to challenge their own idea of themselves as healthy workers.

The case of one participant illustrates some of the problems participants encountered when completing questionnaires and responding to interview questions about illness and sickness. The participant in question flatly denied that he had taken any sickness absence during the period of the study. We reviewed his completed questionnaires together. Here he had indicated days of illness and time off work. The participant explained that this was both true and untrue. He had wanted me to know that he had been ill, so ill in fact that it had affected his ability to work. However, time off work represented periods of 'go slow' and temporary rest. Once symptoms had lessened, he speeded up his work or started work again.

In general, participants' retrospective recollection was of themselves as healthy and committed workers who did not take unnecessary 'sickies'. The data they had provided was evidence of their heroic endeavour, their readiness to work through illness (a theme they had developed in their first interview). As one teleworker put it during the interview, 'I am never off ill. I don't take sickies. Other people do but I have never missed a day off work since working at home. I am a Hercules at work . . . (laughs).' The idea of being a victim who succumbs to illness ran counter to this account.

It became increasingly clear that different accounts were being generated for different purposes. Discussion about the questionnaire data suggested that the formal production of a written record encouraged reports of work undertaken with no time off for sickness. Such evidence alone would serve to confirm ideas of teleworkers as healthy and hard-working employees, often found in the telework literature. Interview data, in contrast, produced more complex perspectives of telework, in which teleworkers described trading opportunities to take time off with illness for the advantages of being able to manage their own illness events and to continue to work at home, as unwonted sickness absence did not undermine their record as healthy, trustworthy employees.

The research suggested that the use of one or other methodology could easily produce a unidimensional picture of the health implications of telework. Combining them offered a complex and constantly negotiated situation in which telework might offer a win–win situation to teleworkers and their employers in managing illness and sickness. Such an interpretation is attractive to business and government policy makers at a time when there is a drive to reduce absenteeism from work. Yet the data also showed that poor health no longer offered a legitimate reason to take sickness leave and that illness incidents are increasingly denied or ignored. The relationship between the two forms of data generated by participants provided the catalyst to identifying these effects.

REFLECTIONS: HANDLING CONTRADICTORY ACCOUNTS

Some researchers (Brannan, 1992; Cresswell, 1994; Greene *et al.*, 1989) recommend the use of qualitative and quantitative methodologies together, suggesting that their strengths combine to make a better study and that each can counterbalance the weaknesses of the other. However, this is potentially problematic. Quantitative and qualitative methodologies demonstrate the clear distinction between reductionist and critical realist/relativist positions in research.

My expectation that the data sets would complement each other was quickly dashed. The preliminary analyses I made, based on the initial interview and quantitative analysis of the five questionnaires, were often refuted by participants in the follow-up interviews. In part, the generation of these different accounts may reflect the perennial problem of validity in questionnaires. I realised that the questions generated different and often very unexpected responses from the subjects. Asking participants for estimates of days off sick was to fail to recognise that on the basis of their lived experience teleworkers differentiated between being unwell and being sick. However, it was by comparing responses gathered by interview with those gathered by questionnaire that this theme emerged with some clarity.

If there were problems at an individual level in combining the analysis of questionnaire and interview data, these problems increased at the final stage. The often contradictory evidence created headaches for the task of reporting the results. In qualitative research there is often a debate about the extent to which what people say represents what they actually do. Different methodologies seek to understand how people tell stories, what they include and omit, and how stories can be constructed and reconstructed from experience. In this research I built up over time several layers of evidence from different methods of enquiry.

My investigation revealed differences between the stories people told face to face and those written as answers in a questionnaire. Participants' responses seemed to be shaped by whether questions had been delivered in written or verbal form. All of us are familiar with this in everyday life: how we respond to a magazine questionnaire on our attitudes may well be quite different from what we'd say to a friend or colleague. Writing a response creates one representation of the answer. It may not, and in this research often did not, match verbal responses.

When questionnaire data were discussed with participants, they described being conscious of providing hard evidence. They reported making more careful calculations of how they responded, spending more time and thought deciding on an answer. They described being conscious of a reader who would regard their written responses as enduring evidence. This suggests that participants were generally unaware of the close scrutiny applied to interview transcripts. There was a sense that written data would convey a different, perhaps more trustworthy, record of events.

Participants were also unsure, despite reassurances on the informed consent form and in discussion, that no one else would see any of the raw data. They were particularly concerned about whether employers would have access to the data. Several participants argued that they should present their work in a good light 'just in case' someone saw their individual results. Others stressed that when writing a work record they wanted me to see their work and endeavour in a good light. A written response seemed to represent a formal audit of work, not an informal record or description.

It was when the two sets of data were brought together for analysis that these incompatibilities became apparent. There was no possibility of triangulation based on confirming themes. Rather, telework experiences seemed to be described for two different audiences and for two different reasons. My use of mixed methodologies had provided an opportunity to see these multiple perspectives and alternative constructions. This struck me as an outcome more valuable than simply confirming the veracity of evidence, as suggested in the process of triangulation (Denzin, 1989).

The research showed the importance, and associated problems, of taking evidence and preliminary analyses back to participants. Each teleworker was sent a draft analysis of their interview and questionnaire data prior to the second interview. Participant validation was chosen over simple member checking, since the latter only involves the person in confirming the accuracy of the record. Participant validation was seen as a means of strengthening the ethics of the study. It allowed participants to be active in the interpretation and presentation of the research and to have face-to-face discussion with me. However, the second round of interviews failed to clarify why there were differences between the quantitative and qualitative evidence. It added yet more data for analysis, as participants shared new ideas and thoughts generated by the previous data.

The construction of life stories is in continuous flux. The coherence of a life story changes with new evidence and experience. My participants and I were involved in a never-ending reinterpretation of their work and health life. This represented what they said, what I said they said, what they said about what I said about what they said and so on! The question was where to stop. Which account would finally gain supremacy? There were multiple perspectives from each participant, derived from the mixed methodology and from an engagement in the research extending over a long period. A report does allow some separation of these accounts. It can present, first of all, what the participants said. It can express what the researcher has to say about the participants' responses. It can also reach conclusions that embody the final sense the researcher has made of the project. Yet beneath this apparent simplicity lies the challenge of finding out how to separate these various accounts.

Each element of my study informed subsequent interpretations. The questions I had asked in interviews shaped the way participants understood and responded to the questionnaire. The process worked in reverse in the case of the second interview. Many participants said they had never been asked about their teleworking lives or about their perceptions and experiences of illness. They therefore had few ready or practised stories to draw on. The requirement to complete a diary of their work, domestic and leisure, calculate time spent on each and respond to closed questions on aspects of telework practice offered participants an unusual opportunity to explore, over the five questionnaires, a number of different aspects of their working lives that had emerged as key themes from the first interviews. This generated new narratives and reflections on their initial stories that greatly contributed to the final analysis.

It seemed to me that in challenging the contradictory accounts provided by the questionnaires and the interviews, participants revealed even more sharply the differences between the various accounts of what they were doing and how it was differently constructed for different audiences and in different forms of verbal or written reports. A mixed methodological approach served to highlight the complexity and ambivalence about working in this way. It showed how individuals generate information about themselves and their employment in many different, often irreconcilable ways.

Participant validation poorly describes this process. Rather than consolidating a shared version of what teleworkers do and experience, the second interviews developed a third story. It was therefore in the discussion that the tensions between accounts were explored and evaluated, and in the conclusions that my analyses of telework developed. The mixed methodology created the seemingly contradictory accounts that participants strove to explain. No consensus emerged, just another fascinating account of teleworking.

My research, in the end, proved to be predominantly qualitative. The demographic and descriptive data provided by the quantitative questionnaires was invaluable to enable me to grapple with the way individuals formulated aspects of their work. It showed the different constructions of this reality and the different meanings for each participant in the final interview. Mixing the two methodologies uncovered different dimensions of a confused and varied employment experience. It revealed some of the ways teleworkers are striving to make sense of this experience, and to manage and safeguard their health.

While these findings are significant, this research experience has reinforced my view that mixing qualitative and quantitative paradigms in one study is hugely problematic. For both the researcher and the participants it involved a mind shift from discussing perceptions and experiences in the messy form that our lives are normally constructed, to making these same experiences factual and numerical. Combining phenomenological data analysis with inferential statistics involves an impossible mind shift. However, I would suggest that exploring how people quantified the aspects of their lives they had already identified as important added an additional dimension to the shared understanding of telework by the participants and myself. Gathering two types of account of the work experience and looking at how these differed was a challenge, but resulted in fuller and richer findings. In the end, the descriptive statistical data offered evidence that would not have emerged from qualitative study alone. In this research project, where so much was new, explored and unknown, the participants and I shared new insights into their work as a result. They felt they had gained from the process and their work helped me to understand – perhaps another win–win result.

REFERENCES

Ahrentzen, S. (1989) 'A place of peace, prospect, and . . . a P.C.: The home as an office', *Journal of Architectural and Planning Research*, 6(4): 271–88.

Bellaby, P. (1999) *Sick from Work: The Body in Employment*, Aldershot: Ashgate Publications.

Bloor, B. (1983) 'Notes on member validation', in Emerson, R. (ed.), *Contemporary Field Research: A Collection of Readings*, Boston: Little Brown.

Bogdan, R.C. and Biklen, S.K. (1982) *Qualitative Research for Education: An Introduction to Theory and Methods*, Boston: Allyn and Bacon.

Brannan, J. (1992) *Mixing Methods: Qualitative and Quantitative Approaches*, Aldershot: Avebury.

Bryman, A. (1988) *Quantity and Quality in Social Research*, London: Routledge.

Comfort, M. (1997) *Portfolio People*, London: Random House.

Creswell, J.W. (1994) *Research Design: Qualitative and Quantitative Approaches*, London: Sage Publications.

Denzin, N. (1989) *The Research Act: A Theoretical Introduction to Sociological Methods*, 3rd edn, Chicago: Aldine.

Fielding, N. and Schreier, M. (2001) 'On the compatibility between qualitative and quantitative research methods', *Forum for Qualitative Social Research Vol. 2(1)*, accessed online at http://qualitative-research.net/fqs-texte/1–01/1–01hrsg-e.htm, 20 March 2005.

Greene, J.C., Caracelli, V.J. and Graham, W.F. (1989) 'Towards a conceptual framework for mixed methodology evaluation designs', *Educational Evaluation and Policy Analysis*, 11(3): 255–74.

Hammersley, M. (1983) *Reading Ethnographic Research: A Critical Guide*, London: Longman.

Huws, U. (1984) 'New technology homeworkers', *Employment Gazette*, 92: 13–17.

Kelle, U. (2001) 'Sociological explanations between micro and macro and the integration of qualitative and quantitative methods', *Forum for Qualitative Social Research Vol. 2(1)*, accessed at http://qualitative-research.net/fqs-texte/1–01/1–01kelle-e.htm, 20 March 2005.

Kuiken, D. and Miall, D.S. (2001) 'Numerically aided phenomenology: Procedures for investigating categories of experience', *Forum for Qualitative Social Research Vol. 2(1)*, accessed at http://qualitative-research.net/fqs-texte/1–01/1–01kuikenmiall-e.htm, 20 March 2005.

Loos, G.P. (1995) 'Foldback analysis: A method to reduce bias in behavioural health research conducted in cross-cultural settings', *Qualitative Inquiry*, 1: 465–80.

McGrath, P. and Houlihan, M. (1998) 'Conceptualising telework: Modern or postmodern?', in Jackson, P.L. and Van der Wielen, J.M. (eds), *Teleworking: International Perspectives: From Telecommuting to the Virtual Organisation*, London: Routledge.

Pile, S. (1993) 'Human agency and human geography revisited: A critique of new models of the self', *Transactions of the Institute of British Geographers*, 18: 122–39.

Probert, B. and Wacjman, J. (1988) 'Technological change and the future of work', *Journal of Industrial Relations*, September: 432–48.

Qvortrup, L. (1998) 'From teleworking to networking: Definitions and trends', in Jackson, P. and Van de Wielen, J.M. (eds), *Teleworking: International Perspectives: From Telecommuting to the Virtual Organisation*, London: Routledge.

Roe, R.A. (1998) 'Foreword', in Jackson, P. and Van de Wielen, J.M. (eds), *Teleworking: International Perspectives: From Telecommuting to the Virtual Organisation*, London: Routledge.

Seale, C. (1998) *Researching Society and Culture*, London: Sage Publications.

Toffler, A. (1980) *The Third Wave*, New York: Bantam Books.

8

Communication Practices in Physiotherapy: A Conversation Analytic Study

RUTH H. PARRY

The methodology considered in this chapter is one that is increasingly being applied to the study of healthcare and therapeutic interactions. Conversation analysis, henceforth CA, was first developed in the 1960s by sociologists who were influenced by ethnomethodology. Since that time, conversation analysts have 'generated a substantial and cumulative body of empirical findings' (Clayman and Gill, 2004, p. 589). Conversation analysts seek to work according to rigorous standards of evidence, and video or audio recorded data are central to this process. Also central to issues of rigour in CA is an elaborate and rather distinctive conceptual foundation and set of methodological requirements (Clayman and Gill, 2004; Peräkylä, 1997).

This chapter begins with a brief introduction to these methodological issues. It then illustrates the procedures of CA and the sorts of findings it can produce, by examining some aspects of research I conducted on physiotherapist–patient interaction. I argue that several features of CA's approach to rigour are highly relevant to other forms of qualitative research, and raise issues that all qualitative researchers should consider seriously. One feature relates to the process of privileging one particular interpretation over others and how this should be done. A second relates to the presentation of clear empirical evidence alongside analysis and claims.

Qualitative Research for Allied Health Professionals: Challenging Choices. Edited by Linda Finlay and Claire Ballinger. Copyright 2006 by John Wiley & Sons Ltd. ISBN 0-470-01963-8.

METHODOLOGY: CONCEPTUAL FOUNDATIONS OF CA

CA is an observational methodology through which detailed descriptions and understandings of social interaction are developed. The term 'conversation analysis' is something of a misnomer, because although its field of interest encompasses 'everyday' conversations, it also includes institutional interactions such as those between patients and health care workers, and interactions between people and technologies such as computers. Also, it can be applied to studying body movements, not just talk. Some of its features, such as its close examination of individual cases, inductive logic, and search for and analysis of 'deviant' cases, are characteristic of qualitative methodologies. However, analyses can also include quantification (e.g. Booth and Perkins, 1999; Peräkylä, 1998). Efforts at quantification are fairly restricted because it is recognised that considerable problems are entailed in trying to quantify communication conduct, and that doing so is often premature (Schegloff, 1993).

CA has its intellectual base within ethnomethodology – the study of the common-sense reasoning, knowledge and procedures by means of which people make sense of each other's actions and of their circumstances, and by which they shape their actions (Heritage, 1987; ten Have, 2004). Conversation analysts aim to describe and explain the detailed organisation of interpersonal communication through fine-grained analysis of recorded interactions. I work in what is broadly termed institutional CA (Heritage, 1997; Drew and Heritage, 1992), which tends to differ from studies of so-called ordinary conversation. The latter often focus on highly general practices and organisations of practice, such as those that govern turn taking, repair and so on. CA studies of institutional interactions tend to focus on how these basic practices are deployed, adapted and specialised in institutional settings.

One way to convey the character of CA is to note some similarities between it and the work of eighteenth-century naturalists (Clayman and Gill, 2004; Heritage, 1988, p. 131). For instance, a naturalist interested in bee dances would observe and 'collect' as many specimens of such dances as possible. These would probably be drawn and described with pencil and paper. (Nowadays, video recordings provide a much better way of forming such collections.) The naturalist would then work to develop systematic and comprehensive descriptions of bee dances. These descriptions would include their characteristic actions, sequences of actions and overall structure, and encompass the range and variations of these. The naturalist would also seek to describe clearly the environments in which dances occurred, what preceded and followed them, and hence what could logically be inferred about their functions and consequences. Similarly, conversation analysts seek to collect a broad range of specimens of the interactional phenomena under study (Peräkylä, 1997): for example episodes in which physiotherapists instruct patients in movements. Importantly, these data are naturally occurring rather than 'made up' or experimentally provoked. Analysts then use inductive logic to identify and describe recurrent patterns of actions, their environments of occurrence, their interactional functions and consequences.

Notice that the naturalist made no attempt to interview the bees about what they thought they were doing! Similarly, conversation analysts use direct observations rather than interviews to come to understandings about 'what is going on' in particular situations and interactions. One reason for this is that practitioners' statements 'routinely gloss over or conceal the practical world' involved in accomplishing occupational goals (Heritage, 1987, p. 262). Clinicians' and patients' accounts cannot be expected to provide comprehensive reports about their complex practices during therapy. Indeed, this is one of my main reasons for choosing a CA approach to studying physiotherapy communication. Additional and very important considerations underlying conversation analytic caution pertain to an understanding that, rather than 'evaluating interview data as more or less accurate reports of external reality, we are obliged to view them as occasions when individuals feel called upon to give accounts of their actions, feelings, opinions etc. For example, the interview may be experienced as an occasion at which to display adequate patienthood or competent professionalism' (Murphy et al., 1998, p. 120; see also Murphy and Dingwall, 2003, Chapter 5). Interviews (and indeed accounts and reports in general) perform actions such as defending, justifying and explaining conduct. Thus the relations between what people do, what they say and what they think are indirect ones (Silverman, 1998, p. 114).

Readers wishing to understand the theory and practice of CA in depth may find the following publications useful: Clayman and Gill (2004) offer a succinct and comprehensive introduction; ten Have (1999) is a key practical textbook; Heath (1997) introduces how CA analyses body movement; Heritage has written extensively about both CA theory and CA practice (e.g. 1995, 1997); Schegloff (1992, 1997) addresses some fundamental conceptual and theoretical issues.

Seminal CA studies within healthcare can be found in Atkinson and Heritage (1984) and Heritage and Maynard (forthcoming). The discussion of CA methodology that follows is limited to a few points of particular relevance to the arguments and illustrations presented in this chapter.

First, the availability of recordings both for analysis and presentations can allow for high levels of validity and reliability in CA work (Peräkylä, 1997; Jordan and Henderson, 1995). Multiple and complex elements of interaction can be analysed and there is access to a level of detail unavailable in other approaches to data collection. Both video and audio recordings have the advantage that they can be made available for scrutiny by others. This makes it easier to check the validity and rigour of original analyses, and to enable others to extend or refute them (Heath and Luff, 1993). Furthermore, when conversation analysts make claims about 'what is going on', they aim only to do so on the basis of what participants themselves display as meaningful, relevant and consequential in their interactions, hence privileging participants' rather than analysts' interpretations (Schegloff, 1992). This is analytically feasible because of the sequential nature of communication: the way that utterances (and nonverbal actions) are connected to each other in sequences 'so that what one participant says and does is generated by, and dependent upon, what the other has said and done' (Drew *et al.*, 2001, p. 59). This sequential structure is a key resource by which we (whether participants or analysts) understand the meanings of what is going on – because each utterance 'inherently embodies and displays its producer's interpretation of the prior actions in the sequence' (Heritage, 1990, p. 28).

As a simple example, imagine a therapist asking a recumbent patient: 'Can you sit up?' If the patient says no, the analyst (and the therapist) can perceive that this utterance has been treated as a question; if the patient moves into a sitting position, it can be seen that it has been treated as an instruction. Soon, I will demonstrate sequential analysis of a couple of extracts from my data. I present the transcripts alongside these so that you can judge the extent to which I have succeeded in privileging the meanings, understandings and orientations that are visible and hearable in therapists' and patients' conduct. One further implication of sequentiality is that communication is understood to be a collaborative accomplishment, and thus it is not adequate to pick out and examine only one party's actions – for example, those of the therapist – in isolation.

DOING THE RESEARCH

My research focuses on communication between health care practitioners and patients. In the study to which I refer in this chapter, I applied a conversation analytic approach to video recordings of physiotherapy treatment sessions with stroke patients. Prior to this research, I had conducted a qualitative interview study with stroke patients and physiotherapists. That work raised questions about what actually happened during treatment, and that is one of the reasons that I went on to examine recordings of real-life physiotherapy, rather than what people say about it. I recorded 72 treatment sessions in four hospitals; 11 senior physiotherapists took part, and 21 (non-aphasic) stroke patients. While I had in mind some specific questions raised by my interview study, I chose to approach my video data with a very broad initial question: 'How do physiotherapists and stroke patients communicate about treatment activities during physiotherapy sessions?' Such a broad question allowed a flexible development of focus, and facilitated emergence of themes shaped by examining the data, rather than predetermined solely by my prior ideas and interests. The rest of this section describes some of the practical choices made and processes involved in the research.

SAMPLE SIZE AND SELECTION

As with other qualitative methods, CA offers no simple equation or algorithm to determine sample size and selection. Some of the considerations that influenced my choices follow. In selecting sites and participants, a balance was struck between homogeneity and variety of data. I aimed to have a large enough set of recordings, involving circumstances that were related but not identical, in order to reliably identify various recurrent patterns of conduct and variations therein. A degree of uniformity was afforded by recording only inpatient rehabilitation treatment sessions, patients who could speak and understand some English, and relatively senior therapists. To help ensure a range of circumstances that arise during inpatient rehabilitation for stroke were captured, I recorded ten therapists, included patients who were at various stages of rehabilitation, and recorded patients and therapists several times at four sites. These strategies enhanced the potential for findings to have validity beyond the specific settings. There were also various practical considerations for instance geographical proximity.

/ Rather than number of **participants** or **recordings**, the number of **interaction episodes** relating to the topic of interest is best thought of as the sample size. So, for instance, hundreds of cases of therapists and patients dealing with patients' errors of movement were available.

EFFECTS OF RECORDING ON CONDUCT

Potential participants often raise concerns that recording interactions could change those interactions to such a degree that they would not reflect everyday practice. I tend to broach this issue proactively, partly because of the ubiquity of the concern, and also because it demonstrates to potential participants that I am aware of and have thought about this issue. Doubtless the presence of recording equipment does influence participants' conduct. Unfortunately, there is no way that any such effects can be precisely verified: one cannot observe the consequences of presence/absence of observation without some sort of observation process – the Observer's Paradox (see ten Have, 1999). Potential effects of recording, and ways of addressing these, can nevertheless be considered in several ways. First, it is thought that the camera influences different aspects of conduct differentially, with verbal actions affected more than physical ones, and content of talk more than its structural organisation. Microbehaviours such as gaze and body movements are also thought to be more strongly affected (Clayman and Gill, 2004; Jordan and Henderson, 1995). Also, it is thought that people habituate to the presence of a camera quite rapidly, especially if certain procedures are followed (Jordan and Henderson, 1995; Heath and Luff, 1993). Details of the specific procedures I used can be found in Parry (2001). One can also argue that if physiotherapy gets done, then whatever it is that participants do in order to accomplish physiotherapy **is** being done. Finally, one should remember that it is not that unusual for therapy to be observed – for example, by patients' caregivers or by students.

ETHICAL APPROVAL

Video data clearly constitute personal data, and the fact that analysis relies on these raw data rather than anonymised, coded information means that care is needed in setting out and explaining the ethical issues involved. In this sort of research, it is often very useful to be able to show data in an undisguised form, as features such as facial expression and gaze direction are essential elements of communication. I have presented 'undisguised' extracts at conferences and workshops for professional audiences. However, for materials that will be publicly accessible, disguising facial and other identifying features is of course essential. In general, it is important to ensure that participants' information makes it clear who will see the data, for what purposes and in what circumstances. Because use of video data in health care research is not very common and well-established guidelines do not exist, ethics committees may feel particularly 'nervous' about this sort of work. I have found it useful to cite guidelines produced by the General Medical Council (2002) and the Royal College of Psychiatrists (1998) (although these mainly address teaching and clinical issues rather than research).

THE PROCESS OF ANALYSING

Once the challenging stages of access and ethical approval are completed, data collection for CA studies is rapid when compared with, say, ethnographic participant observation or longitudinal interview studies. However, analysis is tremendously time consuming (Clayman and Gill, 2004; Peräkylä, 1997). Once I had collected my data, I spent several weeks watching and making brief descriptive written logs of all 72 episodes. At this point I began to make some collections – clips from different recordings, edited together. These were necessarily rather unfocused. I made some early collections on the basis of my own initial interests; some on the basis of the foci of previous studies; and also a rather general tape of 'noticings' (ten Have, 1999, p. 107) – events that just seemed striking or unusual.

Thereafter, systematic, disciplined procedures were used to build data-based analyses. These included selecting a small number of sessions for complete transcription of talk and body movements. The chosen sessions contained most or all elements of treatment that appeared from initial watching to be typical and recurrent. They included patients at various stages of rehabilitation, with different forms of impairments. It took approximately one minute to fully transcribe one second of video data, so limits had to be set on how much could be done. Nevertheless, the very detailed transcripts proved an invaluable resource. Gradually, through watching, reflecting, studying related literature and examining data in the company of experienced researchers, several key themes began to emerge. More systematic and comprehensive collections on these themes were then made. Familiarity with the whole dataset from initial watching and logging allowed comprehensive, systematic searching for relevant episodes. A free-todownload computer program called Transana (Fassnacht and Woods, 2005) is an excellently designed and easy-to-use tool for supporting viewing and/or listening to data, transcribing and making collections using conversation analysis.

TRANSCRIPTION

Transcripts are understood as an important analytic tool, but not as constituting primary data. Transcription allows a clearer and more detailed view of data, and often reveals elements that have been overlooked during inspection of tapes. Also, transcripts can form a resource for presenting relatively 'raw' data within publications and presentations. I used Jefferson's standardised system for CA transcription of verbal activity (Drew and Heritage, 1992, p. 30–1). This system is designed as a compromise between preserving details of talk as it is actually produced (including intonation, silences, overlaps), while remaining simple enough to produce accessible transcripts (Clayman and Gill, 2004). The widespread use of a single system within CA makes for accessibility and contributes to cumulative findings and reliability (Peräkylä, 1997). Methods for transcribing body movements are less well developed (though see Jordan and Henderson, 1995 and Heath, 1997 for examples). Transcripts I present here are simplified and mainly concern verbal elements; nonverbal elements are in italicised script. The conventions used here are shown in Table 8.1.

Table 8.1 Conventions used in transcripts

Symbol	Explanation
[	Indicates the onset of overlapping talk
]	Indicates the end of overlapping talk
(0.0)	Indicates elapsed time in silence in tenths of a second
(.)	Indicates a gap of no more than one tenth of a second
<u>word</u>	Indicates stress on word(s) via pitch or amplitude
:	Indicates prolongation of the immediately prior sound, length of row of colons indicates length of the prolongation
WORD	Indicates especially loud sounds relative to surrounding talk
↑ ↓	Up arrow indicates higher pitch of the following word/syllable, down arrow indicates lower pitch
-	Horizontal dash indicates that the word or word fragment sounds abruptly 'cut off'
(word)	Indicates possible hearing of what was said

FINDINGS: A RECURRENT PRACTICE AND A DEVIANT CASE

One of the three areas of communication on which I eventually focused was communication about successes and shortcomings of performance of treatment activities (Parry, 2004a). Each of the recorded sessions included episodes relating to these matters, hence hundreds of episodes were available for analysis. These numerous episodes allowed me to identify both very common and very unusual patterns in the data. This form of analysis is not always possible in CA; for instance, I was only able to identify eight episodes of treatment goal setting in my data, limiting the sorts of claims I could make about this area (Parry, 2004b).

When extracts are presented, it is important for the reader to be able to understand why the author has chosen this particular extract, and thus what is being claimed with regard to it. The first extract provides a clear and brief example of something that happens very often in the recorded sessions. I therefore use it as an exemplar of a pattern that I claim occurs recurrently. The second extract illustrates some practices that are very unusual in the data. I discuss how and why the extract is unusual, and through it show some of the ways in which deviant cases can enrich analysis.

COMMUNICATING ABOUT SUCCESSFUL PERFORMANCE OF A TREATMENT ACTIVITY: RECURRENT PRACTICES

As this extract begins, the therapist is sitting in front of the patient, who is in the midst of practising moving from sitting to standing.

Extract 8.1

```
T       go on you can do it (.) there yer go
        (0.3)
T       OK (.) lovely ((patient has reached standing position))
P       good
T       yeah that felt alright [there's] no leaning to me so that's good
P                              [yes  ]
T       and then do then doing exactly the reverse as you go down
P                                      ^
                    starts to bend at hips
```

The therapist's talk as the patient nears completion and then completes the activity is clearly positive (lines 1, 3) and the patient acknowledges these comments (line 4). The therapist's positive assessment is soon followed by an instruction to perform a next activity (line 7). The form of the therapist's positive comments, and the rapid progress to the next activity, are typical of such episodes in the recorded sessions. In some, though by no means all, episodes, the therapist elaborates on her general positive assessment by indicating the criteria by which performance is being judged (as in line 5). The patient agrees with the therapist and rapidly responds to her instruction, beginning the movement to sitting by bending her hips (line 8) before the therapist's talk at line 7 is complete.

Notice that I inevitably rely to a degree on common-sense cultural knowledge within my analysis, for instance inferring that 'OK lovely' is positive – although I also use the patient's response (line 4) in making this judgement. Notice the frequent references made to line numbers, so as to empirically ground descriptions and claims and help you to scrutinise them.

Extract 8.2 features a patient who implies disagreement with a therapist's positive assessment and challenges it. Such a response is rarely seen in these data and throws into relief patterns of patients' conduct that are more typical.

COMMUNICATION ABOUT SUCCESSFUL PERFORMANCE OF A TREATMENT ACTIVITY: A DEVIANT CASE

This patient has been undergoing rehabilitation for over three months for a left-sided stroke. He has been diagnosed with post-stroke depression. The therapist told me that rehabilitation had been difficult and that the patient was regarded as 'unmotivated'. In this sequence, he is walking with a tripod stick in his right hand. The therapist supports his affected side, assisting leg movements. A junior physiotherapist pushes a wheelchair behind him, ready in case he should need to sit down.

Extract 8.2

T	this is ↑e<u>x</u>cellent
P	↓is ↓it
	(3.5)
P	((*sniff*)) (.) are you trying to encourage me are ye
	(0.5)
T	wa- what do <u>you</u> think
P	<u>yes</u>
	(2)

T   normally you have <u>two</u> people helping you to ↓walk
P   do I
T   *gazes to patient's face, at end of pause, lowers her head and gaze*
     (3.5)
P   well ↑one is sup<u>por</u>ted by (a) ↑stick
     (0.2)
T   *bending down to reach towards patient's left foot*

T   yeah↑ (.) but there's <u>still</u>: (it's) <u>two</u> people ↑<u>and</u> a stick normally
T   isn't it so:: ↑LEFT LEG then↑ or are you going to do your right
                    ((*patient then steps on right leg, and then continues to
                                                   walk with assistance*))

The therapist produces a positive assessment of the patient's ongoing walking performance that is typically direct and straightforward. She elaborates the criteria by which the performance is judged: 'normally you have two people helping you to walk'. The therapist's talk at line 9 implies not just current success, but overall progression in the patient's abilities because only one person is assisting him to walk, as opposed to the previous requirement of two to support and assist him. This implication of overall progress is a frequent element of evaluations elsewhere in my data.

Unusually for these data, however, the patient implies nonalignment and disagreement. First, he responds to the therapist's 'this is excellent' with 'is it'. Far more frequently, patients respond to assessments in ways that indicate they are received as news, for example 'really?' 'good' (as in Extract 8.1 line 4) and generally provide for a sense that the assessment is taken as good news. But this example is different in that the tone and form of the patient's talk, and particularly his subsequent utterances, for example line 4, convey that he does not treat the assessment as good news. Further, both at lines 10 and 13 he avoids expressing agreement; instead he appears to question the therapist's assessment and explicitly questions the therapist's reasons for giving her assessment: '((*sniff*)) are you trying to encourage me are ye'. In doing so, he questions the motivation underlying her assessment and hence implies doubt as to its truthfulness.

Examination of the sequence indeed shows that the therapist treats his response as implying doubt. After seeking elaboration of his perspective, to which only a minimal response is forthcoming, her next action is to produce the grounds for her positive assessment: 'normally you have two people helping you to walk'. The patient's response, 'do

I', again indicates questioning rather than agreement. During most of the relatively long pause that follows, the therapist gazes at the patient, indicating to him that further talk from him would be relevant (Goodwin, 1979). Towards the end of the pause she briefly glances down, and at this point the patient upgrades his response, producing an assessment that implies a different, and disagreeing, interpretation of his performance and progress. He says, 'well one is supported by (a) stick'. The delay at line 12 and his 'well' mark this response as disagreeing (Pomerantz, 1984). Although the meaning is difficult to discern from the transcript alone, his tone suggests he is referring to the fact that one side of his body is supported by a stick (rather than referring to himself as 'one') – and indeed this is the meaning the therapist seems to make of it in her response at line 16. By emphasising the support of the stick on one side, he counters the therapist's implication of 'excellent' walking performance owing to a reduction in support. Explicit nonalignment with the therapist's assessment through questioning and production of alternative assessments is very rare in these data. In contrast to this episode, patients generally orient towards not questioning or challenging therapists' authority and judgement.

Now turning to how the therapist deals with this situation: as I mentioned, her initial response to the patient's nonalignment is to pursue agreement by elaborating her assessment (line 9), providing information about the basis for her assertion. This is a generic conversational practice used when persons have different versions of events (Pomerantz, 1984). Also, provision of evidence is one strategy by which doctors manage incongruence between patients and themselves (Peräkylä, 1998). When it becomes evident across several turns that the patient is not going to agree, the therapist shifts the topic and the activity at hand, thereby preventing further open dispute (Greatbatch and Dingwall, 1989). She does so through producing a relatively long turn (lines 16–17), whose structure and design limit opportunities for the patient to produce responses and thus further 'negative' talk.

Notice that within the above analysis I drew on other research findings to add detail and to strengthen claims. I was proposing that certain practices seen in these data constitute instances of use of practices whose functioning has been systematically examined in previous research. In doing so, I can strengthen my claims about the functions of these practices in my data.

In general terms, examining this deviant case made it all the more noticeable to me how brief most sequences involving positive assessments are, and how they rely on a mutual orientation towards the therapist's authority. The case also stimulated an interest in what 'being unmotivated' means: in other words, it encouraged me to see and to treat it as an interactional practice – or rather a set of interactional practices – and to start to examine what those might be. Further investigation would be needed, but this case suggests that these practices include delayed responses to therapists' assessments, and disagreements (explicit or implied) with therapists' positive assessments of performance and progress. Also, although the transcript I presented is not sufficiently extensive to show this, this patient's physical responses to instructions are much slower than is usual within the data. So this deviant case allowed me to broaden description of one area of practice (communication about success of performance); it made the regular pattern all the more clear; and it provided insights into the distinctive activity of 'being unmotivated' and into the strategies therapists use to deal with patients' expressed nonalignment. Indeed, the search for and analysis of deviant cases forms an important way by which descriptions and proposals inductively generated in CA are tested for their validity and elaborated (Peräkylä, 1997).

Inevitably, the examples here provide a selective illustration of analysis from a CA perspective. One aspect not particularly evident is the way that analysis moves from detailed descriptions of practices to examining **why** people communicate as they do; that is, to exploration of 'the role which the organisation that has been discovered plays in the communicative and social matrix of interaction' (Heritage, 1988, p. 131). For examples see Parry (2004a) and Peräkylä (1998).

REFLECTIONS

Having conducted research using a variety of methods, I have found in CA a satisfying, constructive research methodology with firm foundations. CA, for me, is a distinctive approach, offering a rigorous methodology and methods, carefully warranted and constructive analysis, and production of practice-relevant understandings and knowledge.

In terms of rigour, a key feature of CA is the availability of detailed relatively raw data both to the analyst and to those inspecting analytic claims. However the most important feature, and one that separates CA from most other qualitative methods, relates to the way claims are warranted. CA takes a principled and restrictive approach to interpretation. It privileges participants' meanings by confining claims to what is visible and hearable in the details of the data. It avoids generating claims on the basis of *a priori* assumptions or on a view that the analyst is somehow in a special position to discern 'what is really going on' (Schegloff, 1997; Silverman, 2001; Drew *et al.*, 2001).

In terms of findings, CA studies do not result in blanket recommendations that certain practices should be used rather than others. Instead, they show how any interactional practice will have a range of functions and consequences, which present both advantages and disadvantages. CA's position is that while it can provide information about communication practices to interested parties (e.g. professionals, patients, policy makers), it is for those parties (rather than the analysts) to decide whether or not a particular practice is appropriate (see ten Have, 1999, pp. 184–7). This stance is especially useful for research in medical settings, where interactions have in general attracted highly critical comment from qualitative research (e.g. Stevenson *et al.*, 2000; Thornquist, 1994). The CA approach seems more likely to produce constructive findings because it emphasises informing, rather than condemning, practice (see Peräkylä and Vehviläinen, 2003).

An example from my study illustrates this point: one element of the work involved examining relations between actual practice and written professional recommendations (Parry, forthcoming). For instance, written professional standards direct physiotherapists to communicate with patients in ways that are open, honest and unambiguous (Chartered Society of Physiotherapy, 2005). Yet when dealing with shortcomings and errors of patients' performance of physical treatment activities, therapists' communication practices are frequently indirect and ambiguous. Rather than simply condemn practitioners for failing to conform to recommendations, I was drawn by the CA approach to examine the logic, the 'good interactional reasons' for these patterns. This analysis also provided a logical basis for considering how standards could be made more appropriate and relevant to practice.

Of course, CA cannot provide answers to every sort of research question. As I have already made clear, analysts tend to avoid investigating or making claims about internal cognitions, perceptions, personal motivations and so on. Also, CA cannot be used in situations where recording is precluded by practical, access or ethical difficulties. This includes some long-term processes and, of course, past unrecorded events.

What CA does do is to generate findings about the highly skilled, but tacit, practices entailed in communicating with one another. It provides detailed descriptions of different strategies for performing particular communicative tasks, and understandings about the functions and consequences of different strategies. Additionally, CA can provide clinicians with a strategy for systematically and constructively analysing and understanding their own communication practices and difficulties. CA thus provides practical tools and information. Therapists can use these to enhance their ability to analyse, reflect on and improve their communication.

REFERENCES

Atkinson, J.M. and Heritage, J. (1984) *Structures of Social Action: Studies in Conversational Analysis*, Cambridge: Cambridge University Press.

Booth, S. and Perkins, L. (1999) 'The use of conversation analysis to guide individualized advice to carers and evaluate change in aphasia: A case study', *Aphasiology*, 13(4): 283–303.

Chartered Society of Physiotherapy (2005) *Core Standards*, revd edn, London: Chartered Society of Physiotherapy.

Clayman, S.E. and Gill, V.T. (2004) 'Conversation analysis', in Hardy, M. and Bryman, A. (eds), *Handbook of Data Analysis*, Beverly Hills: Sage Publications.

Drew, P., Chatwin, J. and Collins, S. (2001) 'Conversation analysis: A method for research into interactions between patients and health-care professionals', *Health Expectations*, 4(1): 58–70.

Drew, P. and Heritage, J. (1992) *Talk at Work: Interaction in Institutional Settings*, Cambridge: Cambridge University Press.

Fassnacht, C. and Woods, D. (2005) Transana v2.04, Madison, WI: The Board of Regents of the University of Wisconsin System, accessed at http://www.transana.org, 20 March 2005.

General Medical Council (2002) 'Making and using visual and audio recordings of patients', accessed at http://www.gmc-uk.org/standards/default.htm, 20 March 2005.

Goodwin, C. (1979) 'The interactive construction of a sentence in natural conversation', in Psathas, G. (ed.), *Everyday Language: Studies in Ethnomethodology*, New York: Irvington, pp. 97–121.

Greatbatch, D. and Dingwall, R. (1989) 'Selective Facilitation: some preliminary observations on a strategy used by divorce mediators', *Law and Society Review*, 23(4): 613–41.

ten Have, P. (1999) *Doing Conversation Analysis: A Practical Guide*, London: Sage Publications.

ten Have, P. (2004) *Understanding Qualitative Research and Ethnomethodology*. London: Sage Publications.

Heath, C. (1997) 'The analysis of activities in face to face interaction using video', in Silverman, D. (ed.), *Qualitative Research: Theory, Method and Practice*, London: Sage Publications, pp. 183–200.

Heath, C. and Luff, P. (1993) 'Explicating face-to-face interaction', in Gilbert, N. (ed.), *Researching Social Life*, London: Sage Publications, pp. 306–26.

Heritage, J. (1987) 'Ethnomethodology', in Giddens, A. and Turner, J. (eds), *Social Theory*, Cambridge: Polity, pp. 224–72.

Heritage, J. (1988) 'Explanations as accounts: A conversation analytic perspective', in Antaki, C. (ed.), *Analysing Everyday Explanation: A Casebook of Methods*, London: Sage Publications, pp. 127–44.

Heritage, J. (1990) 'Interactional accountability: A conversation analytic perspective', in Conein, B., Fornel, M. and Quere, L. (eds), *Les Formes de la Conversation, Vol. 1*, Paris: CNET, pp. 23–49.

Heritage, J. (1995) 'Conversations analysis: Methodological aspects', in Quasthoff, U.M. (ed.), *Aspects of Oral Communication*, Berlin: Walter de Gruyter, pp. 391–418.

Heritage, J. (1997) 'Conversation analysis and institutional talk', in Silverman, D. (ed.), *Qualitative Research: Theory, Method and Practice*, London: Sage Publications, pp. 161–82.

Heritage, J. and Maynard, D.W. (forthcoming) *Practising Medicine: Talk and Action in Primary Care Encounters*, Cambridge: Cambridge University Press.

Jordan, B. and Henderson, A. (1995) 'Interaction analysis: Foundations and practice', *Journal of the Learning Sciences*, 4(1): 39–103.

Murphy, E. and Dingwall, R. (2003) *Qualitative Methods and Health Policy Research*, New York: Aldine de Gruyter.

Murphy, E., Dingwall, R., Greatbatch, D., Parker, S. and Watson, P. (1998) 'Qualitative research methods in health technology assessment: A review of the literature', Health Technology Assessment, NHS R&D HTA Programme, NCCHTA, University of Southampton, Southampton, accessed at http://www.ncchta.org, 20 March 2005.

Parry, R.H. (2001) 'Communication between stroke patients and physiotherapists', PhD thesis, University of Nottingham, British Library reference DXN054515.

Parry, R.H. (2004a) 'The interactional management of patients' physical incompetence: A conversation analytic study of physiotherapy interactions', *Sociology of Health and Illness*, 26(7): 976–1007.

Parry, R.H. (2004b) 'Communication during goal setting in physiotherapy treatment sessions', *Clinical Rehabilitation*, 18(9): 668–82.

Parry, R.H. (forthcoming) 'Professional recommendations and actual practice in physiotherapy: Managing troubles of physical performance', *Communication and Medicine*.

Peräkylä, A. (1997) 'Reliability and validity in research based on tapes and transcripts', in Silverman, D. (ed.), *Qualitative Research: Theory, Methods and Practices*, London: Sage Publications, pp. 201–19.

Peräkylä, A. (1998) 'Authority and accountability: The delivery of diagnosis in primary health care', *Social Psychology Quarterly*, 61(4): 301–20.

Peräkylä, A. and Vehviläinen, S. (2003) 'Conversation analysis and professional stocks of interactional knowledge', *Discourse and Society*, 14: 727–50.

Pomerantz, A. (1984) 'Agreeing and disagreeing with assessments: Some features of preferred/dispreferred turn shapes', in Atkinson, J.M. and Heritage, J. (eds), *Structures of Social Action*, Cambridge: Cambridge University Press, pp. 57–101.

Royal College of Psychiatrists (1998) 'Guidance for videotaping', London: RCP, accessed at http://www.rcpsych.ac.uk/publications/cr/cr65.htm, 20 March 2005.

Schegloff, E.A. (1992) 'On talk and its institutional occasions', in Drew, P. and Heritage, J. (eds), *Talk at Work: Interactions in Institutional Settings*, Cambridge: Cambridge University Press, pp. 101–34.

Schegloff, E.A. (1993) 'Reflections on quantification in the study of conversation', *Research on Language and Social Interaction*, 26(1): 99–128.

Schegloff, E.A. (1997) 'Whose text? Whose context?', *Discourse and Society*, 8(2): 165–87.

Silverman, D. (1998) 'The quality of qualitative health research: The open-ended interview and its alternatives', *Social Sciences in Health*, 4(2): 104–18.

Silverman, D. (2001) *Interpreting Qualitative Data: Methods for Analysing Talk, Text and Interaction*, 2nd edn, London: Sage Publications.

Stevenson, F.A., Barry, C.A., Britten, N., Barber, N. and Bradley, C.P. (2000) 'Doctor–patient communication about drugs: The evidence for shared decision making', *Social Science and Medicine*, 50(6): 829–40.

Thornquist, E. (1994) 'Profession and life: Separate worlds', *Social Science and Medicine*, 39(5): 701–13.

9

Using Biographical Research with Disabled Young People

MICHAEL CURTIN

Research investigating the effect of impairment on disabled young people is wide ranging and substantial. However, most of this research is from an adult perspective. It explores the problem from the point of view of professionals involved in the care of disabled young people, of the parents of such young people, and of disabled adults reflecting back on their childhood. Researchers have generally ignored the views and opinions of disabled young people themselves, and as a result their voices have often not been heard (Barnes, 1996; Morris, 1997; Shakespeare and Watson, 1998; Kitchin, 2000). Disabled young people's voices are largely absent from debates on the major issues that influence their lives, such as inclusive education (Pitt and Curtin, 2004). This is because the welfare–protectionist approach to raising young people is more commonly used than the empowerment or participation approach (Flekkøy and Kaufman, 1997; Burr and Montgomery, 2003). The welfare–protectionist approach argues that young people are not physically, cognitively and emotionally ready and able to participate competently in decisions about their lives.

I began to question the relevance of adult voices speaking on behalf of disabled young people because these were not the views of disabled young people. Even where disabled adults reflect back on their childhoods, their perspective is unavoidably coloured by hindsight, the passing of time and their experiences.

Qualitative Research for Allied Health Professionals: Challenging Choices. Edited by Linda Finlay and Claire Ballinger.   Copyright 2006 by John Wiley & Sons Ltd.   ISBN 0-470-01963-8.

I became interested in knowing what disabled young people thought about their lives while they were still young. This became important as I realised just how little I knew about so many of the disabled young people I had worked with, apart from what was related to the therapy I was offering. I began searching for a means of discovering what they thought about their lives and how they felt about their impairment. I wanted to find a more direct way of studying disabled young people that would allow their voices to be heard. One way that appealed strongly to me was to work collaboratively with them to write their biographies.

In this chapter, I describe the approach I used to investigate the life stories of nine young people who had a motor impairment. I provide a brief summary of the findings I made on the basis of these stories, together with my reflection on the collaborative nature of the research. Various aspects of the research process are illustrated with extracts from my research diary to identify my thinking on issues that arose as I gathered and analysed the data.

After completing this research, I found it interesting to reflect on how I had felt when I began interviewing the participants. The entries in my research diary show that I doubted my ability to conduct this type of research. This lack of confidence was demonstrated by my timidity in making contact with the young people who had agreed to be involved in the study.

I am still very nervous about this research. I feel that it will be worthwhile, but I am not sure that I am the right person for the job. I will be able to do it, but will I do it well? I guess the only way is to immerse myself in it, to continually be reflective and to be open-minded to the possibilities . . . I am a bit timid when it comes to following up the expression of interests shown by the parents. I kid myself that it is because I do not want to cause someone an inconvenience, which I dare say is partly true. I think the main reason, though, is that I fear rejection. I fear being told that my research is a waste of time. As long as I don't have to hear this, I feel there is always hope.

METHODOLOGY

In order to elicit the voices of disabled young people and to hear their views and opinions, biographical research methods were used to gather their life stories. Biographical research focuses on a person's life experiences (Erben, 1998). This type of research is concerned with individuality, the dynamics of change and how knowledge is culturally and historically situated (Sparkes, 1994; Preece, 1996). It allows research participants to describe their experiences in their own words and ascribe their own personal meaning to those experiences (Pollock *et al.*, 1997). Atkinson and Walmsley (1999) argue that among methodologies biographical research has the greatest potential for self-representation. Narrating their life story not only represents a way in which people can make sense of their life; it also enables them to claim a self-identity (Frank, 2000; Habermas and Bluck, 2000).

Biographical research is particularly appropriate for investigating disability issues because it offers 'counter-narratives' to dominant narratives. It is a way of reconstructing alternative realities from the viewpoint of marginalised groups (Thomas, 1999).

DOING THE RESEARCH

RECRUITMENT

Nine disabled young people, aged between 10 and 13 years, were involved in this study. They were recruited via staff at two special needs schools, who sent research information packs to parents of appropriate disabled young people. Nine parents expressed interest in learning more about the study. I discussed the research in more detail with these parents and their disabled children to ensure that they knew what was involved before they committed themselves to further interviews.

Generally, seeking parental permission is considered to be the proper way to access young people in Britain. Young people are rarely free to decide entirely by themselves whether to participate in research (Masson, 2004). Masson (2004) points out that there are usually several adult gatekeepers who control access to young people. Within my research, the gatekeepers were the staff at the schools and the parents of the young people approached. Such gatekeepers have the responsibility to protect young people in their care and to check out the motives of those who want access to the young people. Going through gatekeepers involved handing over some control of the recruitment process to others. At times, this handing over of control caused concern. I felt that once the information packs were handed over to the two schools, there was very little that I could do to ensure an appropriate number of respondents. I became anxious about whether I would receive the number of responses I had hoped for. In my research diary I wrote:

I regularly visited my post tray but it was void of any returns. I became quite anxious about the lack of response and wondered why parents did not want their children to be involved in the research. My thoughts wandered from the irrational, 'I wonder what they're hiding?', to the more reasonable and logical, 'My child is doing enough things and this is not really necessary at the moment'. When I put myself in the shoes of the parents, I probably would do the same.

As I was planning to work with the young people to write their life stories, I had to be sure that they were choosing to be involved in the research of their own accord, rather than because their teachers and parents thought it would be a good idea. This is in line with the move for young people to be considered active participants who have a right to say what they will be involved in (Prout and James, 1997; Burr and Montgomery, 2003). At my initial meetings with the families I therefore tried to engage the disabled young person in as much conversation as possible to ensure that they understood what the research was about and what would be expected of them. I gave each of them a research information sheet, which contained the same information as the parent information sheet but in slightly simpler language. At the end of the meetings, each disabled young person was given the option to be involved in the research. All nine young people and their parents agreed to be involved. This was then formalised by the parents and the young people completing and signing a research consent form. Once the young person and a parent completed their respective consent forms, an appointment was made for the first interview.

In spite of my efforts to ensure that the young people were free to choose whether or not to be involved in the research project, I was not convinced that they were truly free. Part of my concern was that the young people's gatekeepers – their parents and staff – may, intentionally or unintentionally, have put pressure on them to agree to be involved. I did what I could to provide a free choice for the young people, but in the end I was not sure how free they felt to express their true opinion. One participant, Ronald, was of particular concern to me. He agreed to be involved but never really got engaged with my questions during any of the interviews. I reflected on his case in several diary entries. The extract that follows was written following my last interview with him:

As Ronald suggested that I could see him at home during the holidays I took him up on the offer . . . I have to confess, however, to being a little pissed off with the visit and feeling that it was a complete waste of time.

It confirmed my suspicion that Ronald did not really want to be involved in the research and that he did not have the communication or social skills with which to engage in the research effectively . . . When I arrived at his house . . . he was playing football on the Playstation. Although his mum asked him to stop playing, he took his time to switch it off . . . However, rather than switch it off and focus on our conversation (which was very one way in that I tried to stimulate a conversation and Ronald was basically monosyllabic in his replies) he left the television on and watched a black and white war movie the whole time I was there. He rarely turned to talk to me and gave the impression that he was not very interested in me being there. Anyway, that was my last interview with Ronald. I have to admit that I am a wee bit glad, as he has not really been engaged . . . I will have to reflect on what I can learn from my experiences with Ronald rather than look upon it as negative.

DATA-GATHERING TOOL AND PROCEDURE

Interviews were used to collect the participants' life stories, as this method was considered appropriate for discovering young people's perceptions of their experiences of their social and physical worlds (Ginsburg, 1997). Kitchin (2000) argues that rich data can be accessed through interviews as interviewees can express and contextualise their feelings. This supports the contemporary emphasis on narrative and biographical research approaches in the construction of knowledge and understanding of marginalised voices, such as those of disabled young people (Leicester and Lovell, 1997). The interviews were relatively open ended, unstructured and nondirective, allowing each disabled young person to lead. Significance was attached to the way each of them reported, presented and made sense of their lives (Frank, 2002). To ensure that the interviews were conducted at an appropriate level, Bowden's (1995) guide for communicating with young people was loosely followed.

Bowden (1995) states that prior to interviewing, researchers need to build a trusting and workable relationship with young interviewees. This can be difficult for adults researching young people due to their perceived position of authority, so spending time on building rapport prior to any interviews was essential (Kitchin, 2000). My initial informal meeting with the parents and young people was part of the process of building a relationship. Where possible, before and after each interview I allowed time to talk with each young person, their parents and siblings, about things not necessarily related to the research. I also actively listened to what the young people were saying (Lloyd-Smith and Tarr, 2000; Curtin, 2001) and trusted their version of events, demonstrating this by not clarifying various factual details with parents or school staff. I found this difficult, as it became clear at several stages that the information the young people told me was factually incorrect or might have repercussions for them and their family of which they were unaware. I pondered this problem at various times during the research, as these diary entries show:

> I am also concerned about how I will know if the children are telling me the correct things. Part of me wants to be able to clarify issues with the parents. However, if I do this then I am no longer telling the story from the child's perspective . . .
>
> I have the urge when I am writing the children's stories to change some things particularly related to the family. Like Xanthe doesn't really mention her younger sister except to say that she is a pain. I have to control my urge and try and write what is there but it is difficult. In the end it needs to be their decision what goes in, what is left out and how it is presented . . .
>
> Today . . . Simon was talking quite positively about his father and tended not to mention his mother very much at all. This made me feel awkward because most of my dealings have been with his mother and I guess I am a little prejudiced against his father . . . I have no substance on which to base my opinions or assumptions. It was just an initial impression, a few tit-bits that I have been told and I guess the gut feeling that I think his mother has been wronged. But as I know none of the history which led to the separation, it is irresponsible for me to think such thoughts. Still my awkwardness remains, because if I print what Simon has said today, I am wondering whether it will have some type of negative impact for either of his parents.

Bowden (1995) suggests that for a young person to be placed in a position of expertise and therefore be able to engage actively in the research, the interviews must be structured around themes that are familiar. The interviewer must not display too much prior knowledge as this may intimidate the young person. In addition, the interviewer must become skilled at asking appropriate open questions, as young people generally do not respond well to direct questions (Dockrell et al., 2000).

The disabled young people involved in my study were placed in the position of experts because the topic for the interviews was their life stories (Curtin, 2001). Each interview was relatively unstructured so that the participants could focus on what they saw as important. I began the first interview with an open question, loosely based on Wengraf's (2001) suggestion that participants be asked to speak freely about their lives. The disabled young people responded to this open-ended question in various ways. All but two required some guidance on what to talk about. I provided this guidance by repeatedly adding questions and statements such as 'Talk about things that have been important to you in your life' or 'What are your earliest memories?' and 'Anything else?' I needed to add these prompts to encourage the disabled young people to talk more fully about their lives and to help them engage in the interviews.

As the research was geared to gathering biographical information, each participant was interviewed several times to ensure that as much material as possible was collected. The young people were informed that the interviews would stop when they felt they had told me all they wanted to. In each interview, they were always asked if there was anything else that they remembered about their life that they would like to talk about. Other questions encouraged them to expand on what they had previously said. In this way, the focus of each interview was negotiated at the beginning and, where necessary, at appropriate intervals during its course. Each disabled young person was interviewed up to four times within a four-month period. After this there was a break to allow time for me to complete all the transcripts and write a first draft of their biographies.

The completed first drafts of the biographies were next sent to the disabled young people for their comments. Follow-up interviews were conducted, where the focus was on correcting the first drafts of the biographies and adding further information that the young people wanted to include. For all the participants apart from one, this follow-up interview was the final one. They were generally happy with their biographies, pending the changes and additions that were discussed in the interview.

However, one participant, Simon, wanted to add more information so requested more interviews. I saw him a further five times. I was pleased that Simon wanted more interviews as I felt that he had not shared very much information prior to the break. He had spoken predominantly about his interest in the Eurovision Song Contest and the Children in Need event, but said very little about his life. The first draft of his biography was very short and appeared to be lacking in substance. I was even considering dropping Simon from the research. But my diary entry following the fifth interview with Simon indicated a change of focus in the topics he was willing to talk about:

Did I have a bit of a breakthrough with Simon today or was it a false alarm and nothing to get too excited about? This was the first interview in which he did not mention Children in Need or Eurovision. And it was the first interview where he appeared to start to tell me something about his family. He did not cut me off like he did in the past when I asked him about his parents' separation, he actually talked a little about it.

Despite this, Simon was still reluctant to go into any depth about his life story and in the end I just had to accept what he wanted to tell me:

These interviews with Simon are interesting. I am not sure why he likes me coming out to see him but he really does. Not that that means he tells me about his life. In fact, I seem to be noticing that he is quite adept at not telling me any of the information that I would like to hear. Every time I asked a question about his life – even one as quite basic as 'Tell me about your life, what are the things that you remember, what are the things that are important to you?' Simon will inevitably change the subject and I guess talk about something that he is more comfortable with.

Following the final interviews, a second draft of each biography was completed and sent to the participants to ensure that the stories were a valid representation of what they had told me about their lives.

ANALYSING THE DATA

There were several stages to the data analysis. The first stage involved completing the transcripts of all the interviews conducted in the initial four-month period. The second stage was to read and reread each transcript to achieve some insight into the biography of the young person involved. On this basis, the transcripts were gently reworked and edited so that they became the first draft of the young person's biography. This was done by reproducing as far as possible the exact words the young person had used in the interviews. I occasionally put in linking words but, as much as possible, I made a point of using only the participants' own words. When the first drafts of the biographies were completed, they were sent to each disabled young person for further comment.

The third stage of analysis was the follow-up interview with each young person after they had read the first draft of their biographies. This generally involved an extended interview in which amendments and corrections were noted and additional material was added. This stage was completed when each young person indicated that they had said all that they wanted to say.

The fourth stage involved the full transcription of the final interviews and, on this basis, the production of the second draft of the biographies. Amendments and corrections were made and additional material inserted. The second drafts were returned to the young people for their comments and corrections. When each young person was satisfied with the second draft, the final drafts were written and used for the next stage of analysis. The final stage of analysis involved the identification and interpretation of the dominant themes in each young person's biography, using a thematic field analysis (Wengraf, 2001). Chase (1996) states that aspects of the interviewees' stories may be presented thematically and be supplemented by the researcher's analysis identifying how each young person described and evaluated their experiences.

I was concerned about how to present the biographies and themes. I felt an obligation to write in a way that would be meaningful for the young people who had shared aspects of their life with me. I wrote in my diary:

> I am also thinking about how I can do my best for these participants. I have promised them all a book about their lives based on the stories that they tell me. I want to make these books individual and original. It is a chance for me to practise some creative writing and perhaps to see if I have what it takes to write in different ways . . .
>
> One thing that I have become aware of after these visits is the responsibility that I have undertaken to ensure that I do the biographies justice. I felt that the parents were trusting me with their children's stories . . . I have been given something precious and . . . I must do my best to be respectful and to ensure that I do a good job. I would intensely dislike it if I upset the parents and/or the children. In some ways, this may affect how I present the biographies.

I wanted to write in an accessible way. After all, the concept of an academic publication was foreign to all my participants. I considered Richardson's (2000) suggestion that researchers should experiment with writing, because it is a way of analysing and engaging with texts at greater depth and is also a means to reaching a diverse audience. Although I am yet to explore alternative genres of writing, I have considered contributing pieces to more popular journals and writing short stories and poems aimed at challenging young people's awareness and understanding of disabled people. Using a variety of methods to present and publish the life stories of the disabled young people involved in my study would, I thought, be a way of making my research more accessible to them. It might also enable the research to reach a wider audience and have a greater impact.

FINDINGS: A BRIEF OVERVIEW

My aim in conducting this research was to focus on the individuality of the nine disabled young people as depicted through their personal life stories. My belief was that disabled young people should not be defined by their impairment. Rather, they should be considered first and foremost as people. Although the interviews were nondirective and open ended, allowing each young person to talk about their life in a way they found comfortable, all the participants talked about their family, friends and education and set out their views on having an impairment. Each presented their life experiences from their own unique perspective.

On the whole, the young people indicated that their parents were very supportive, providing them with opportunities to experience life as fully as possible. Relationships with siblings were described as 'normal' in the sense that the young people did not feel themselves to be treated differently because of their impairments. Crucially, some recognised that they at times supported their nondisabled siblings, a factor that has been overlooked in previous research. The extended family also played an important role by accepting the disabled family member, offering everyday experiences and helping with medical and therapy interventions.

All the young people considered friendships to be important. Those who attended a special needs school generally felt comfortable interacting with peers who also had impairments. They preferred mixing with peers who understood them and did not treat them as different. The remaining participants, who attended mainstream schools, had mixed views about who they preferred to mix with. Some liked to be friends only with nondisabled peers, while others preferred friendships with disabled peers. These differences seemed to relate, in part, to the personalities of the young people. What was important to them was their inclusion in a peer group that they wanted to be with. One interesting finding from the stories was that putting disabled young people together did not necessarily mean that they would become friends.

Those young people attending a special needs school spoke positively of their segregated education. They felt that they were understood by both the staff and the other pupils, that their needs were provided for and that they were given plenty of opportunities to be active. Those going to a mainstream school had experiences that ranged from feeling fully included to feeling totally excluded. A number of factors appeared to play a role in shaping their experience, including the attitudes of the staff and students and the general systems in place at their particular school. The young people took a variety of positions within the inclusion–segregation debate.

In spite of the difficulties that some of the young people had experienced, they were relatively positive about their life. They did not see having an impairment as a tragedy; they just got on with life. They were reasonably positive about the medical interventions they had experienced, indicating that the functional improvements they achieved made such interventions worthwhile. They regarded themselves as ordinary, except for the fact that they used a wheelchair for mobility.

The positive outlook of the young people in this study lends support to the idea of developing an affirmation model of disability. This proposes that having an impairment can be a positive experience, and can result in a life that is rich in satisfaction and a sense of self-worth (Swain and French, 2000).

This study has highlighted that disabled young people sharing the same medical label have differing needs, aspirations, opinions, attitudes and emotional states, and that all of these are as complex as those of nondisabled young people (Lewis and Kellet, 2004). Considering, indeed emphasising, the individuality of disabled young people highlights the issue of participation and the right of such young people both to express their views and opinions and to be listened to (Kirby and Woodhead, 2003).

REFLECTIONS

When I reflect on this particular research, the main issue I wrestle with is my failure to achieve the degree of collaboration with the disabled young people that I had wanted. While I was able to achieve a degree of collaboration in the production of each biography, the young people were not involved in the analysis of their stories and therefore I did not clarify the themes with them. This was partly due to the deadlines I was trying to meet. But I was also unsure about how to involve the young people in analysis of this type. This failure of mine raised the issue of representation, and led me to question whether it was my voice or their voice that had taken precedence. I accepted that the main responsibility for the final content and layout of each biography was mine and acknowledged that I might have misrepresented or suppressed the very voices I was attempting to make heard. Stanley (1993) and Richardson (2000) argue that as it is not possible to exclude the researcher's voice from the text, the construction of a biography should be a collaborative effort between the researcher and the participant.

It has become clear to me that if the voices of disabled young people are to be heard more clearly, the collaborative method used in my study requires further development. Arvay (2003) proposes using a collaborative narrative method to make the relationship between the researcher and the participants equal, as a way of dealing with issues around voice and representation. She engages her participants both in the production of their biography and in the analysis of the data. However, it is worth noting that her use of the collaborative narrative method has been exclusively with adults. For me, the challenge remains one of how to engage disabled young people in the interpretation process. Strategies to enable this to happen require careful thought.

In my study, none of my participants challenged the content, layout or presentation of their stories, even though they were encouraged to do so. While they were ready to correct spellings, grammar and the occasional factual error, they seemed reluctant to engage with the research at a deeper level. To work more collaboratively with these young people would mean demanding from them a greater commitment of both time and effort. Building the necessary rapport would take time and would require the young people to have a greater understanding of the research. Perhaps they would need to be involved at the development stage. This degree of collaboration has the potential to ensure that the final stories are truly representative of young people's voices. This is the challenge I embrace as I contemplate future biographical research with disabled young people.

In conclusion, I have provided an overview of my biographical research investigating the life stories of nine disabled young people. I offered an outline of the research, including a rationale of the methodology, an explanation of the method and a summary of the findings. I then reflected on how I could develop this research to facilitate a more collaborative relationship with disabled young people. In spite of my initial lack of confidence in my ability to manage this kind of research, the journey I have made while investigating the life stories of young people with motor impairment has been worthwhile. I have become convinced that biographical research methods have the ability to challenge stereotyped and ill-informed attitudes held by society and contribute to a greater understanding of disabled young people.

REFERENCES

Arvay, M. (2003) 'Doing reflexivity: A collaborative, narrative approach', in Finlay, L. and Gough, B. (eds), *Reflexivity: A Practical Guide for Researchers in Health and Social Sciences*, Oxford: Blackwell Science.

Atkinson, D. and Walmsley, J. (1999) 'Using autobiographical approaches with people with learning difficulties', *Disability and Society*, 14(2): 203–16.

Barnes, C. (1996) 'Disability and the myth of the independent researcher', *Disability and Society*, 11(1): 107–10.

Bowden, S. (1995) 'Development of a research tool to enable children to describe their engagement in occupation', *Journal of Occupational Science: Australia*, 2(3): 115–23.

Burr, R. and Montgomery, H. (2003) 'Children and rights', in Woodhead, M. and Montgomery, H. (eds), *Understanding Childhood: An Interdisciplinary Approach*, Chichester: Open University and John Wiley & Sons Ltd.

Chase, S. (1996) 'Personal vulnerability and interpretive authority in narrative research', in Josselson, R. (ed.), *Ethics and Process in the Narrative Study of Lives*, Thousand Oaks, CA: Sage Publications.

Curtin, C. (2001) 'Eliciting children's voices in qualitative research', *American Journal of Occupational Therapy*, 55(3): 295–302.

Dockrell, J., Lewis, A. and Lindsay, G. (2000) 'Researching children's perspectives: A psychological dimension', in Lewis, A. and Lindsay, G. (eds), *Researching Children's Perspectives*, Buckingham: Open University Press.

Erben, M. (1998) 'Biography and research method', in Erben, M. (ed.), *Biography and Education: A Reader*, London: Falmer Press.

Flekkøy, M. and Kaufman, N. (1997) *The Participation Rights of the Child: Rights and Responsibilities in Family and Society*, London: Jessica Kingsley Publishers.

Frank, A. (2000) 'The standpoint of storyteller', *Qualitative Health Research*, 10(3): 354–65.

Frank, A. (2002) 'Why study people's stories? Dialogical ethics of narrative analysis', *International Journal of Qualitative Methods*, 1(1), Article 6, accessed online at www.ualberta.ca/~ijqm/english/engframeset.html, 20 March 2005.

Ginsburg, H. (1997) *Entering the Child's Mind: The Clinical Interview in Psychological Research and Practice*, Cambridge: Cambridge University Press.

Habermas, T. and Bluck, S. (2000) 'Getting a life: The emergence of the life story in adolescence', *Psychological Bulletin*, 126(5): 748–69.

Kirby, P. and Woodhead, M. (2003) 'Children's participation in society', in Montgomery, H., Burr, R. and Woodhead, M. (eds), *Changing Childhoods: Local and Global*, Chichester: Open University and John Wiley & Sons Ltd.

Kitchin, R. (2000) 'The researched opinions on research: Disabled people and disability research', *Disability and Society*, 15(1): 25–47.

Leicester, M. and Lovell, T. (1997) 'Disability voice: Educational experience and disability', *Disability and Society*, 12(1): 111–18.

Lewis, V. and Kellet, M. (2004) 'Disability', in Fraser, S., Lewis, V., Ding, S., Kellet, M. and Robinson, C. (eds), *Doing Research with Children and Young People*, London: Sage Publications.

Lloyd-Smith, M. and Tarr, J. (2000) 'Researching children's perspectives: A sociological dimension', in Lewis, A. and Lindsay, G. (eds), *Researching Children's Perspectives*, Buckingham: Open University Press.

Masson, J. (2004) 'The legal context', in Fraser, S., Lewis, V., Ding, S., Kellet, M. and Robinson, C. (eds), *Doing Research with Children and Young People*, London: Sage Publications.

Morris, J. (1997) 'Gone missing? Disabled children living away from their families', *Disability and Society*, 12(2): 241–58.

Pitt, V. and Curtin, M. (2004) 'Integration versus segregation: The experiences of a group of disabled students moving from mainstream schools into special needs further education', *Disability and Society*, 19(4): 387–401.

Pollock, N., Stewart, D., Law, M., Sahagian-Whalen, S., Harvey, S. and Toal, C. (1997) 'The meaning of play for young people with physical disabilities', *Canadian Journal of Occupational Therapy*, 64(1): 25–31.

Preece, J. (1996) 'Class and disability: Influences on learning expectations', *Disability and Society*, 11(2): 191–204.

Prout, A. and James, A. (1997) *Constructing and Reconstructing Childhood*, London: Falmer.

Richardson, L. (2000) 'Writing: A method of inquiry', in Denzin, N. and Lincoln, Y. (eds), *Handbook of Qualitative Research*, 2nd edn, Thousand Oaks, CA: Sage Publications.

Shakespeare, T. and Watson, N. (1998) 'Theoretical perspectives on research with disabled children', in Robinson, C. and Stalker, K. (eds), *Growing Up with Disability*, London: Jessica Kingsley Publishers.

Sparkes, A. (1994) 'Life histories and the issue of voice', *International Journal of Qualitative Studies in Education*, 7(2): 165–83.

Stanley, L. (1993) 'On auto/biography in sociology', *Sociology*, 27(1): 41–52.

Swain, J. and French, S. (2000) 'Towards an affirmation model of disability', *Disability and Society*, 15(4): 569–82.

Thomas, C. (1999) *Female Forms: Experiencing and Understanding Disability*, Buckingham: Open University Press.

Wengraf, T. (2001) *Qualitative Research Interviewing: Biographic Narrative and Semi-Structured Methods*, London: Sage Publications.

10

Low Back Pain: Exploring the Meaning of Exercise Management through Interpretative Phenomenological Analysis (IPA)

SARAH G. DEAN, JONATHAN A. SMITH AND
SHEILA PAYNE

Interpretative phenomenological analysis (IPA) is a qualitative methodology with considerable potential for research in therapy-related settings. Emerging from the discipline of health psychology, IPA lends itself to researchers who, like me (SD), wish to explore the lived experience of individuals undergoing health care.

While doing research on patient adherence for my MSc degree, I had found that quantitative approaches provided only limited insights and understanding. There was, I was sure, more to the patients' stories than could be captured through the statistical analysis of structured questionnaire data. However, as qualitative research was unexplored territory for me, I was unclear as to which qualitative methodology to pursue. IPA appealed in three ways. First, its focus on individual experiences seemed to allow people to tell their own story, something that

Qualitative Research for Allied Health Professionals: Challenging Choices. Edited by Linda Finlay and Claire Ballinger.   Copyright 2006 by John Wiley & Sons Ltd.   ISBN 0-470-01963-8.

was lacking in my earlier quantitative approach. Secondly, it explicitly acknowledges the importance of the researcher's interpretation. This was especially important to me, as I felt unable to divorce myself from the knowledge I had gained through previous research and clinical experience and IPA accepts this. Thirdly, IPA's practical, step-by-step procedure and clear guidelines (see Smith, 1995) appealed to my preference for a practical, 'doing' approach to work – an approach that might be considered typical of many physiotherapists!

For therapists, especially those new to qualitative methods, who are engaged in qualitative research requiring in-depth analysis of an individual's experiences, IPA offers exciting possibilities. The example of IPA in action presented in this chapter stems from one aspect of a research study I conducted in a physiotherapy setting as part of my PhD (Dean *et al.*, in press). The chapter focuses on two elements of the qualitative research processes inherent within IPA: verification and layered analysis.

Jonathan, as the main proponent of IPA, was the adviser for the methodology and Sheila, as one of my PhD supervisors, has extensive experience in qualitative health research. Throughout this chapter I will highlight their involvement in the work.

METHODOLOGY

Discussion with my supervisor, Sheila, confirmed that using a qualitative approach would require a different way of thinking about research. At the time I did not realise the extent to which my thinking would be challenged by this change in approach. I started by reading various texts and research articles. I read about epistemology and explored accounts of research conducted in qualitative health psychology, medical sociology, medical anthropology and studies using ethnography. I returned to these publications a number of times, but never more so than during the interpretative phase of my research. This was when my way of thinking about doing research finally altered. The characterisation of IPA that follows was something I wrote after I had conducted the study. It was only at that point that I felt I had a sufficient grasp of IPA's underlying philosophy to provide a clear account of the methodology.

IPA is linked with the broader field of phenomenology, which emerged in the early twentieth century as a psychological approach to investigating events, occurrences or happenings in the lived world. These are things we all know about but possibly experience in many different ways. It is how this experience is perceived and related through language that is the basis of phenomenological analysis. The experience of the event, the immediate physical context, the social and cultural influences and past experiences of similar events all mean that people may experience a particular event or occurrence in different ways. IPA can also trace its origins to symbolic interactionism (Smith *et al.*, 1997; Smith and Osborn, 2003), whose proponents argue that researchers should focus on the meaning an individual gives to an event or occurrence. Central to symbolic interactionism is the view that the way people perceive an experience is directly reflected in how they talk about it and how they behave in relation to it. Meanings are seen to occur as a result of social interaction: for example that between researcher and participant. It is only through a process of interpretation that these meanings can be understood.

In IPA this interpretative process occurs at different levels (Smith and Osborn, 2003). In the first, participants offer their interpretation of meanings and cognitions through their use of language. This may not always be a straightforward process. Ideas may still be in an undeveloped state, feelings may be difficult to express in words, and thoughts may seem too personal to be disclosed. A second level of interpretation then takes place as the researcher interprets the participant's comments. Here the researcher may not only respond directly to what has been said but also builds a picture of the participant's mental and emotional states, noting how these might influence what they do and do not say. I found this second level of interpretation of the methodology particularly appealing, and it proved one of the determining reasons for my selecting IPA over other qualitative approaches.

In summary, IPA is a methodological approach that draws on several different theoretical perspectives and incorporates them into analysis of the meaning an individual ascribes to their lived experience of particular phenomena. This meaning is made sense of by the process of interpretation, which in turn results from the interaction between the individuals concerned. This chapter reflects the way in which I, as a novice to qualitative research, learned to use IPA. I believe it was not possible for me to be fully conversant with the underpinning methodology before embarking on the study; it was only by doing the research that I got to grips with IPA and found my way of thinking about research fundamentally changed.

DOING THE RESEARCH

DATA COLLECTION

The purpose of my study was to explore patients' perceptions of low back pain (LBP) and exercise in the context of adopting self-management for back care. In the case of LBP, figures suggest that up to 63 per cent of physiotherapy patients may not perform enough of their exercises to obtain therapeutic benefit (Sluijs *et al.*, 1993). It seemed to me that a qualitative approach might be a potentially rich way of exploring adherent behaviour and the meaning of an individual's nonadherence within the setting of physiotherapy for LBP.

As IPA focuses on in-depth interpretation of participants' experiences, it is usual to study only a small number of participants. This was my starting point. Rather than attempting to study a representative group in order to make generalisations, I sought to sample from a well-defined, or homogeneous, group and then analyse individual cases in detail. This allowed me to make specific statements about this particular group of people (see Smith and Osborn, 2003). It was therefore important to describe my participant group clearly, even though some of its characteristics might not be explicitly linked to the analysis. The participants in my study were patients between their first and second session of physiotherapy who were prescribed exercise therapy for their LBP. The group comprised four males and five females between the ages of 28 and 59 years (average of 39.5 years). All had English as their first language, since command of a common language was required for the purposes of successful data collection. Two were white-collar professionals, three were self-employed, two were secretaries (one retired) and two were houseworkers.

The definition of LBP used in my study is that of 'nonspecific intermittent' or recurrent LBP (Waddell, 1998). This definition excluded 'red flag' patients with serious spinal pathologies (Clinical Standards Advisory Group, 1994) and patients with persistent chronic pain requiring multidisciplinary pain clinic interventions. Ethical approval for the research was obtained and through a pilot study links were established with a physiotherapist who set about recruiting the nine participants. The research interviews were conducted in the homes of the participants or at their place of work. Before each interview, I ensured my own safety by notifying someone in an appropriate position about the interview venue and my expected time for returning to the office.

IPA allows for a variety of data collection methods, including case notes, field diaries and patient diaries. In common with most researchers who have so far used IPA, I chose semi-structured interviewing as my principal method of data collection (Smith *et al.*, 1999). Given my familiarity with interviewing patients, it was not necessary for me to learn interviewing skills *per se*. However, I did need to refine my interviewing skills for research purposes. For example, I needed to conduct the interviews on a more exploratory basis, taking care to use open-ended questions and to allow the interviewees to take the lead. I tried to adopt the position of a somewhat naïve listener, one who never put words into the mouths of interviewees or offered answers to questions. I sought to allow pauses and if I offered gentle prompts, I strove to ensure they were not value laden. One prompt that I found particularly useful was 'How do you feel about that?' This indicated that I was interested in the participant's experience but also sensitive to the effect that talking about it might have.

Conducting interviews with such considerations in mind is time consuming. There would be little space for all this in the traditional, time-pressed clinical interview, and my research interviewing technique required practice and feedback. Pilot interviews proved very useful, and I also devoted as much time as possible to developing my schedule of semi-structured interviews (see Smith and Osborn, 2003, for a useful guide). The schedule I designed took up only one side of an A4 sheet of paper, with key questions in bold and prompts indented below. This enabled me to glance at the schedule and quickly recall questions without breaking the flow of conversation. It also allowed for swift changes to the order in which I posed questions, thereby helping me to follow a participant's line of response while ensuring all my key questions were covered. The schedule, which focused on participants' experiences of LBP and their subsequent activity and exercise adherence, was tested during a pilot study involving volunteers. Only minimal refinement to the schedule was found necessary.

Before being interviewed, participants were asked if they had any queries about the study, and I made a point of supplying any information that was requested. Participants then signed the informed consent form.

Each interview began with me checking the participant's details by way of warm-up. I used a Sony Walkman Professional tape recorder with normal tapes and, on Sheila's valuable advice, a good-quality microphone. A sound check was made prior to commencing. The interviews varied in length, lasting between 35 minutes and just under an hour. No participant became distressed at talking about their specific experiences or wished to curtail the interview, and so no referral to support agencies was needed. After recording stopped, the interviewees were thanked. Any comments made after the recorder was switched off (there were several instances when this occurred) were summarised as notes in my field diary immediately after I left the venue. Subsequently I wrote to each participant's general practitioner informing them of their patient's involvement in the study and reassuring them that the necessary consent had been obtained. I also made a point of writing to each participant to thank them for their involvement in the study.

FINDINGS

LAYERED ANALYSIS

Layered analysis begins at an early stage in IPA. In the case of my study, I transcribed the first six interviews. Doing the transcription myself helped me get to know the data. The small number of transcripts made it possible for me to hold a mental picture of my respondents' stories (Smith *et al.*, 1999). For the task of transcribing the remaining interviews I employed a transcription secretary, but then checked the resulting transcripts against the recording. Two such 'check reads' per interview proved necessary as the secretary was not familiar with medical terminology. Establishing a transcript template also proved helpful. I followed the format recommended by Smith (1995), with wide margins, a short line of central text, and line and page numbering. I then assigned each transcript a code to ensure anonymity and confidentiality. The code was an interview number, so that it was possible to track the sequence of interviewing, as well as participant pseudonyms. I then used these names in the transcripts.

For a novice qualitative researcher, one appealing feature of IPA is that the layered analysis follows a relatively structured set of stages (see Smith *et al.*, 1999). I found the analogy of peeling layers off an onion a useful way of characterising what I was attempting to do. The first layer – the outer layer of the onion, if you like – involved me placing interpretative comments and any identified themes in the margins of the first six transcripts. As each line of the transcript was very short, it helped to underline or highlight key words that triggered these comments. The next layer saw me using these comments and themes as the basis of interpretation of the remaining interview transcripts. At this stage I created a new computer document for each theme. In each I briefly described the theme and included all transcript extracts relating to it. Cut and paste computer options made this a relatively simple task, but manual cuttings work equally well if you have enough floor space! In some instances the same interview extract was used to illustrate two or more different themes. Each clip had the assigned code and where possible the original transcript page number.

Despite being predominantly mechanical, these initial stages of analysis – the first two layers of the onion – helped me gain familiarity with the data. My interpretative work was able to proceed at the same time. There then followed a period of theme refinement in which I repeatedly moved themes and the examples around (I used handwritten diagrams on sheets of paper, but a whiteboard works equally well). In this way I reworked the theme descriptions until the heart of the onion was revealed.

VERIFICATION

Once the initial themed documentation was ready, formal verification began. This involved scrutiny of the documentation by an independent researcher; in this case, Jonathan. Jonathan had considerable experience with IPA methodology and, as he had not been involved in the data collection process, he had the necessary independence. In effect he was coming 'fresh' to the data. This verification process was necessary for subsequent evaluations of the research that sought to assess its quality. The nature of qualitative research means that all such assessments are somewhat subjective. However, they do allow an opportunity for reflecting on the work, which is also an integral part of the qualitative analysis process.

In IPA, verification can take place in several stages. In broad terms, it continues the onion peeling analogy. First, the verification process focuses on the initial theme descriptions and examples. It examines how well the research data are represented by the themes. Secondly, it looks at the connections made between interview data and themes. In the case of my research, Jonathan agreed with the connections I had made. Sufficient outer layers had been removed and the onion was ready for cooking.

The analysis could have ended at this point. In IPA terms it would be described as a 'typology of responses' (Smith, 1995, p. 24). This is similar to content analysis, whereby data are collated in a systematic

Table 10.1 Summary of themes emerging from the interviews

Patient interview main themes	Component
Making sense of signs and symptoms	Causal events and activities
	Physical attributions
Matching understanding and expectations	Wanting a diagnosis
	Expectations and satisfaction with physiotherapy treatment
Prioritising time for managing LBP	The importance of a routine
	Self-management versus health care

way and may be presented quantitatively (see Wilkinson, 2003) or descriptively. This level of analysis may be entirely appropriate for the purpose of the research, for example to inform a subsequent quantitative study; to employ mixed methods, with the qualitative study embedded in a quantitative study or because limits need to be placed on the complexity of work as it is being conducted at undergraduate level. In my onion analogy this level of analysis would represent basic preparation for cooking. Table 10.1 provides an example of how this typology of responses could be presented from the findings of my study.

I first wrote up these results by giving theme descriptors, illustrating my analysis with transcript excerpts and discussing my findings in relation to the literature. The first theme comprised two components: causal beliefs and physical attributions. These two components stem from psychological theories, but they did not provide an explicit link to understanding adherence in the case of these participants. I therefore reworked the components into a main theme: 'making sense of signs and symptoms'.

"MAKING SENSE OF SIGNS AND SYMPTOMS"

Patients seek to make sense of their LBP experience by identifying the cause and nature of their problem. This process of making sense of signs and symptoms, also known as attribution theory (see Heider, 1958), is now considered a fairly typical patient phenomenon (Moss-Morris, 1997). Studies of patients with other chronic and nonlife-threatening diseases suggest there is a wide range of internal and external attributions made by patients about their particular condition (Scharloo and Kaptein, 1997). In my study, several patients attributed their LBP to external events or activities: for example a sporting injury or road traffic accident. One patient, however, stated a causal belief that was related to fear of a significant pathology. As Jessica put it, 'Well, I suppose you think, automatic[ally] you think of the cancer.'

Jessica went on to explain that her niece, who had recently died from cancer, had earlier complained of hip and leg pain. Jessica's LBP had produced pain in her leg, so she thought the cause might be 'the cancer'. Such catastrophic beliefs (Kendall *et al.*, 1997) are commented on in the literature as being a predictor of long-term chronic disability for cases in which there is a lack of corresponding significant impairment or pathology (Waddell, 1998). It may be that such beliefs limit adherence to treatments designed to help the patient self-manage since, in this example, cancer would not be treated by exercise therapy.

My second main theme, 'matching understanding and expectations', expanded on the way in which patients make sense of their LBP and makes a more direct link with perceptions of treatment and likely adherence. 'Wanting a diagnosis' was an important element in this theme. Although the participants seldom used the term 'diagnosis', I interpreted some of their comments as seeking a biomedical label for their problem. Having a diagnosis was also seen as the starting point for expectations about their treatment. I therefore grouped it with the second main theme rather than including it within the causal beliefs component of the first theme.

"MATCHING UNDERSTANDING AND EXPECTATIONS"

This theme described the participants' beliefs regarding physiotherapy and its likely outcome. It covered what they expected from treatment and it sought to examine the extent to which these expectations matched what they believed to be the cause of their LBP.

In the first instance, patients 'want a diagnosis' in order to confirm their understanding of LBP. As Jill, one of the participants, put it, 'Yes, in a way I was quite relieved to actually see this bulging disc because I thought, well I haven't imagined it all this time.' As I interpreted it, Jill was telling me that the technical diagnosis (based on her MRI scan result) confirmed the physical cause of her pain. It meant she (and other people) could now believe her pain was real. I interpreted this as evidence that patients believe in, and want, objective, medically based diagnoses. This may, or may not, correspond with their beliefs about the proposed treatment. After all, it may not be clear to Jill how a bulging disc could be helped by exercise therapy. Patients can see the benefits of exercise in general, but they are not certain this will work for them. They have reservations about adhering to the treatment.

Another participant, Mandy, was not able to make a match between her LBP and what she understood physiotherapy could offer. As a result, she intimated that she was unable to believe in the treatment:

> I can't see how physiotherapy is going to, I don't understand how, I'm not saying it won't, I don't understand how it could work. Especially if I have got a bulging disc or something well you're not going to be able to put it back in and it's going to be touching the nerve or whatever. You can't, I don't, I shouldn't imagine you can move the nerve and you can't move the bulging bit . . . Um, as far as the physio's concerned, I need to sort of find out a bit more about, I need it explained a bit more about how it can work for me to have an opinion on that.

Mandy's scepticism suggests the need for a coherent model capable of explaining both the condition and how it can be treated. Patients need to have grasped the model, and expressed some faith in it, before being expected to adhere to treatment. This may be one way to help patients manage their LBP. However, while evidence from technological sources such as scans and X-rays seems to provide patients with confirmation that they are indeed suffering from LBP, patients have yet to accept the medical view that scans and X-rays tell us very little about the origins of LBP. For patients the technical evidence explains the cause and provides a meaningful diagnosis that should correspond to the treatment. If this is congruent with the proposed physiotherapy, I argued that adherence to prescribed exercises will be more likely to occur. Matching patients' perceptions of LBP with their treatment should promote better adherence, but the trick is how to convince patients that biomedical evidence is unlikely to be valid!

The two main themes identified above had areas of overlap and could perhaps have been refined further. I sought to distinguish between patients' lay beliefs (the first theme) and biomedical concepts such as diagnosis and treatment (the second theme). While this represented just one way of analysing the interview data, it seemed to me a fairly straightforward way of managing the data for my 'typology of responses'.

In order to continue with the layered analysis that is typical of IPA and to go beyond this notion of biomedical versus other reasons for nonadherence, I needed to take further steps. Attention at this point in the IPA process related to the interpretation given to the thematic analysis. This required me to devote time to thinking (recording my thoughts on a dictaphone while walking my two dogs was especially productive) and to sharing ideas with Jonathan. Our discussions resulted in changes to theme titles and the reworking of theme descriptors. We worked to ensure that the themes were representative of the participant group and we established a consensus on which extracts best illustrated each theme. At this point I also reflected in detail on my interpretative role and how this could be affecting the analysis. This meant removing yet more layers of the onion, metaphorically speaking, to reveal the core.

Throughout this time I was continually writing notes, jotting memos in my field diary and drafting accounts of the themes. I also attended an IPA workshop and this proved seminal in challenging my thinking. For one thing, it made me far more conscious of the biomedical worldview that was inherent in my thinking. Given my predominantly biomedical training as a physiotherapist and my quantitative research background, this was hardly surprising. I found it stimulating to discuss my work with other IPA researchers and in particular with Mike Osborn, who was doing research involving a chronic pain clinic group (Osborn and Smith, 1998). I would highly recommend making use of such contacts either in person or through the IPA website (http://www.psych.bbk.ac.uk/ipa). I returned to my background reading with renewed vigour and a different perspective. As my thinking changed, I continued to discuss epistemology with Sheila as well as other qualitative health researchers and to set aside time for reading and thinking. I became more and more immersed in the challenge of doing qualitative research.

Layer by layer, the analysis continued. So too did the verification process. This ensured that Jonathan and I agreed on the final interpretative analysis as well as the theme content. The writing-up of the study passed through many drafts. I also sought verification by informally discussing my thematic interpretation with some of my participants.

The following example illustrates the next layer of in-depth analysis that is typical of IPA. The data is taken from the third main theme of my typology of responses, titled 'prioritising time for managing LBP'.

"PRIORITISING TIME FOR MANAGING LBP"

Patients are expected to make time in their day for their LBP exercises, but making time can be a problem. Alan's comments during my interview with him illustrate the problem:

Doing your exercises twice a day or whatever. Finding the time in the morning and find the time in the evening. It's er, you know, that's something I'm, I'm not yet sort of managing to, to do regularly enough I think to, to really make the difference.

Harry, another of my participants, also had difficulty in setting aside time for exercise. As he told me, 'there's always a thousand things that need to be done and somehow doing exercises . . . tends to fall further and further down the list.'

The participants in my study emphasised the importance of establishing a routine. This was revealed by Alan's use of the word 'discipline', implying that he should be in control, should take care of his back, should allow exercise to be part of his normal life:

Eventually I'll sort of get my act together and sort of um, er, absorb it into my lifestyle but it's er, you know, not something I can do overnight. Some people who are very disciplined can probably sort of get it straightaway.

It was at this point in the research that my wider reading became useful. From this I knew that living with pain can interfere 'with the preferred life' (Hansson *et al.*, 2001, p. 294) and that it can interrupt normal life (Eccleston, 2002), with treatment becoming an additional interruption. This explained why it was hardly surprising that people did not adhere to exercise therapy. Minimising the interruption caused by exercising may be one way of tackling the adherence problem. Alan, for example, described his wish to 'absorb' exercises into his lifestyle. I found that the medical sociology literature provided further insights into this notion of interruption. According to constructs of self and social identity (Kelly, 1992), individuals hold a personal model of themselves as fit, independent, busy people with full active lives. This self-image is threatened by LBP. Moreover, having to make time every day to do exercises as part of rehabilitation means acknowledging that the self is weak and disabled. Adhering to treatment regimes means accepting this 'spoilt' identity. In contrast, not adhering means retaining the original self-image. The challenge for physiotherapists is to 'normalise' rather than 'medicalise' LBP, in the process ensuring that patients no longer perceive LBP as interrupting their everyday life, thereby helping patients to see LBP as just part of their everyday existence and to view their exercises as part of their routine.

My reading also showed me, however, that many psychological models fail to take into account the importance of routines or habitual behaviours as explanations for particular types of health behaviour (Bennett and Murphy, 1997, p. 41). My conclusion was that adherence-promoting strategies should focus on facilitating the development of routines. I also concluded that greater success might be achieved by adopting health promotion principles rather than depending on medical models. For example, it might be worthwhile adopting the 'personal trainer' approach when seeking to support people with LBP to engage in exercise programmes.

REFLECTIONS

Research conducted on the basis of IPA routinely includes a section appraising the merits and limitations of the study. Tackling this allowed me to reflect on my interpretation in relation both to the participants and to my analysis of the data. Acknowledging the researcher's interpretation is a key feature of IPA (stemming from its epistemological origins in symbolic interactionism).

Reflecting on my research, I was aware of a number of weaknesses and limitations. For a start, the fact that I was doing my PhD on a part-time basis meant that the interviews were conducted over a long period (about one year), resulting in some loss of momentum. However, this did give me the opportunity to do some layered analysis between interviews. Another weakness was the shortness of some of the interviews and the fact that in some of them the same issues were repeatedly commented on. However, the topic possibly had an inherently limited timespan and longer interviews might not have produced significantly greater insight. This is not to belittle the experiences of patients with LBP. Rather, it suggests that my interest in adherence issues was rather greater than that of my participants! Alternatively my skills, as a novice to this type of interviewing, may have been the limiting factor.

Follow-up interviews may have provided more in-depth information, allowed refinement of my interview technique and helped participants to be more at ease with the process, especially if they perceived me to be an expert in LBP. Participants might also have felt more able to discuss their thoughts and feelings, or to consider issues arising from the first interview. Follow-up interviews could also have given me the opportunity to track my participants' progress through their treatment and to monitor their adherence (or nonadherence).

In conclusion, my study explored experiences of LBP from the perspective of nine patients. The analysis suggested that making sense of LBP is important for patients. For adherence to treatment to occur, a match needs to exist between patients' beliefs about the condition and their beliefs about what can be expected from treatment. The layered analysis made possible by IPA highlighted the importance of prioritising or managing time when seeking to strengthen patients' adherence to treatment. The reiterative verification process ensured that the research reflected the participants' experiences of why exercises might not be undertaken. The interpretative analysis reveals the importance of individual perceptions of treatment and underlines how helping patients to manage time may facilitate adherence.

In this chapter I have presented the theoretical underpinnings of IPA, focused on the importance of verification in qualitative analysis and discussed how IPA affords the opportunity to perform layered analysis. Table 10.2 provides a summary of this process, demonstrating

Table 10.2   The process of IPA in relation to layered analysis and verification

IPA process	Layered analysis	Verification	Analogy
Getting to know your data	Transcription Templates and interview codes and participant pseudonyms	Proofreading	Obtaining the onion
Typology of responses	Notes in margins Early themes Creating Word documents for each theme Cutting and pasting examples	Early themes discussed with independent researcher/adviser Theme titles, descriptions and interview examples agreed	Peeling off outer brown layers
	Present as table. Discussion may be descriptive account in relation to literature with transcript examples		Onion undergoing basic preparation for cooking
Interpretative analysis ↕ (occurs before and during the process of writing up) ↕ Writing up	Numerous rereading Theme refinement Reiterative and reflexive process Interpretation examined Check data examples represent themes and vice versa Requires thinking time, discussion and draft writing Present as in-depth analysis – rich description of theme and data examples. Present separately or integrated into discussion section.	Checking and agreeing interpretation with adviser. Discussion to refine themes: titles and description of themes Checking and agreeing transcript extracts are best examples for each theme Consult with participants (optional)	More layers removed to reveal sweet inner centre of the onion Final, specialised, preparation of the onion

what I believe to be the relatively straightforward step-by-step nature of this methodology and how I have married this with in-depth and reflective interpretation in a robust, trustworthy manner.

As a methodology I regard IPA as a health psychology approach to qualitative health research, and the example used in this chapter indicates how I have applied this to a therapy setting in a meaningful and useful way. I believe it has been an ideal methodology as a training for me in qualitative research as it allowed a gentle introduction to a different way of thinking about research for someone coming from the quantitative, biomedical paradigm. The step-by-step analysis, or onion layers, allowed me to stop at any one point in the process, although the more steps I took the more intriguing it became to remove further layers. The fascinating thing about doing qualitative analysis is that however many layers one removes in achieving an interesting, coherent story, there are always more layers that can be removed. Of course, I have yet to get to the centre of my onion.

REFERENCES

Bennett, P. and Murphy, S. (1997) *Psychology and Health Promotion*, Buckingham: Open University Press.

Clinical Standards Advisory Group (CSAG) (1994) 'Report of a CSAG Committee on Back Pain', London: HMSO.

Dean, S.G., Smith, J.A., Payne, S. and Weinman, J. (in press) 'Managing time: an Interpretative Phenomenological Analysis of patients' and physiotherapists' perceptions of adherence to therapeutic exercise for low back pain', *Disability and Rehabilitation*.

Eccleston, C. (2002) 'Attentional features of a chronic pain presentation: Interruption, worry and the dissolution of identity', Psychology Department Lecture, Spring series, Southampton: University of Southampton.

Hansson, M., Bostrom, C. and Harms-Ringdahl, K. (2001) 'Living with spine-related pain in a changing society: A qualitative study', *Disability and Rehabilitation*, 23(7): 286–95.

Heider, F. (1958) *The Psychology of Interpersonal Relations*, New York: John Wiley & Sons Ltd, cited in Atkinson, R.L., Atkinsonn, R.C., Smith, E.E., Bem, D.J. and Nolen-Hoeksema, S. (eds) (2000) *Hilgard's Introduction to Psychology*, 13th edn, Fort Worth: Harcourt Brace.

Kelly, M. (1992) 'Self, identity and radical surgery', *Sociology of Health and Illness*, 14(3): 390–415.

Kendall, N.A.S., Linton, S.J. and Main, C.J. (1997) 'Guide to assessing psychosocial yellow flags in acute low back pain', Wellington, New Zealand: Accident Rehabilitation and Compensation Insurance Corporation and the National Health Committee.

Moss-Morris, R. (1997) 'The role of illness cognitions and coping in the aetiology and maintenance of chronic fatigue syndrome (CFS)', in Petrie, K.J. and Weinman, J.A. (eds), *Perceptions of Health and Illness*, Amsterdam: Harwood Academic Press.

Osborn, M. and Smith, J.A. (1998) 'The personal experience of chronic benign lower back pain: An interpretative phenomenological analysis', *British Journal of Health Psychology*, 3: 65–83.

Scharloo, M. and Kaptein, A. (1997) 'Measurement of illness perceptions in patients with chronic somatic illnesses: A review', in Petrie, K.J. and Weinman, J.A. (eds), *Perceptions of Health and Illness*, Amsterdam: Harwood Academic Press.

Sluijs, E.M., Kok, G.J. and van der Zee, J. (1993) 'Correlates of exercise compliance in physical therapy', *Physical Therapy*, 73(11): 771–82.

Smith, J.A. (1995) 'Semi-structured interviewing and qualitative analysis', in Smith, J.A., Harre, R. and Van Langenhove, L. (eds), *Rethinking Methods in Psychology*, London: Sage Publications.

Smith, J.A., Flowers, P. and Osborn, P. (1997) 'Interpretative phenomenological analysis and the psychology of health and illness', in Yardley, L. (ed.), *Material Discourses of Health and Illness*, London: Routledge.

Smith, J.A, Jarman, M. and Osborn, M. (1999) 'Doing interpretative phenomenological analysis', in Murray, M. and Chamberlain, K. (eds), *Qualitative Health Psychology*, London: Sage Publications.

Smith, J.A. and Osborn, M. (2003) 'Interpretative phenomenological analysis', in Smith, J.A. (ed.), *Qualitative Psychology: A Practical Guide to Research Methods*, London: Sage Publications.

Waddell, G. (1998) *The Back Pain Revolution*, Edinburgh: Churchill Livingstone.

Wilkinson, S. (2003) 'Focus groups', in Smith, J.A. (ed.), *Qualitative Psychology: A Practical Guide to Research Methods*, London: Sage Publications.

ACKNOWLEDGEMENTS

I would like to thank my PhD supervisor John Weinman, Professor of Psychology as Applied to Medicine, Health Psychology Section, Psychology Department (Guy's) Institute of Psychiatry, King's College London, and the School of Health Professions and Rehabilitation Sciences, University of Southampton, for the support they provided while I completed this study.

APPENDIX

Key to transcription conventions:

. . .   speech omitted
( )   name of participant (changed by author to protect confidentiality)
[ ]   text inserted by author

11

Using a Biographic-Narrative-Interpretive Method: Exploring Motivation in Mental Health

TANYA CAMPBELL-BREEN AND FIONA POLAND

Understanding the concept of motivation is central to the therapeutic relationship between client and health care professional. Mental health professional practice continues to rely, perhaps surprisingly, on concepts of client (patient) motivation that are based mainly on adherence to medical interventions (Maclean *et al.*, 2000) and pharmacological treatment (Wong and Van Tol, 2003). While evidence suggests that intrinsic (internal) as well as extrinsic (external) factors are relevant to conceptualising motivation, the positivist emphasis of research methodologies in this field perhaps limits the adequate inclusion of internal factors in favour of external ones.

Such a broader, client-centred perspective is not often evident in current clinical research on motivation. Qualitative research methodologies offer a way of addressing this lack of balance. In the case of our own research, we opted for a hermeneutic, narrative approach to study motivation in mental health. This approach, with its emphasis on individual experiences, offered a different way of viewing motivation – one that recognised a wider temporal frame beyond the illness context. The approach was consistent with our surmise that clients' life stories may represent valuable meaning making about their motivation, and that they draw on their whole life experience. Such narratives, we thought, could therefore incorporate an individual's interpretation of their past

Qualitative Research for Allied Health Professionals: Challenging Choices. Edited by Linda Finlay and Claire Ballinger.   Copyright 2006 by John Wiley & Sons Ltd.   ISBN 0-470-01963-8.

in the light of their current and future expectations. Motivation cannot be appreciated unless parts of the life story as well as the whole are included in the interpretive process. Adopting a hermeneutic approach would help us show how motivation cannot be understood only in the context of illness or single experiences. Broader life experiences may provide additional insights into client motivation in mental health practice.

The biographic-narrative-interpretive method (BNIM) offers an especially systematic yet open approach to the study of motivation. It challenges researchers' assumptions and perhaps, too, the ways health professionals conceptualise client motivational status. However, using BNIM raises a number of challenges. Some of these will be explored in this chapter, which draws on a single example from Tanya's (Campbell-Breen, 2004) hermeneutic, narrative study of motivation.

This chapter is structured in four main sections. First, we explain the reasoning for our methodological approach to the study of motivation, explaining how the data collection and analysis of the BNIM enhance the rigour of our study. Second, we discuss how dealing with gate-keepers in recruiting clients seen as vulnerable can raise particular challenges for this type of research. Third, we look at how this type of analysis worked in developing findings for a single client case. In the final section, we present some reflections on using this approach in the study of motivation.

METHODOLOGY

A HERMENEUTIC, NARRATIVE APPROACH

Research on motivation theory, based largely in the field of psychology (Sewards and Sewards, 2003), is predominately focused on medically derived theoretical frameworks. Where studies have taken a narrative approach to client experiences, these have either been limited to the illness experience or predetermined by professional theoretical frames. We therefore saw a need to take into account the views and experiences revealed through the client's own construction of the meaning of their own lives. This meant finding an approach that would prioritise client accounts and set limits on the researcher's capacity to structure such accounts in ways that could be less meaningful for the client.

The study drawn on here aimed to explore motivation in mental health by deriving meaning from what participants 'say' rather than what they are observed 'to do'. By focusing on individuals' stories or narratives of their experiences, research places importance on meaning as constructed in narrative (Denzin, 2000). Hermeneutic philosophy is based on the tradition of oral histories understood in the context of meaning and action (Grondin, 2002). This provides a framework in which individual lives can be understood, a 'hermeneutic circle' of interpretation in which the parts can be understood in light of the whole and vice versa (Heidegger, 1967). One area of 'life experience' in which BNIM methodology has produced powerful results is in the study comparing the accounts of both victims and perpetrators of the Holocaust (Rosenthal, 1998).

Other narrative theorists suggest that meaning cannot be derived from stories that do not follow expected narrative structures. However, while we concede that not all mental health clients are able to construct stories that readily conform to such structures, we would argue that clinicians are ready to appreciate client experience based on how they tell their stories. Just because clients have mental illnesses and construct various types of stories does not mean that we are not able to construe or appreciate their motivation. Researchers who make use of narrative approaches are often challenged about the 'truthfulness' of the accounts they collect. However, we suggest that even if the events and experiences mentioned in client stories are 'fabricated', this forms part of the way that participants construct their own stories – whether intentional or unintentional. Narrative approaches place less analytic emphasis on what is 'real' than on what is said. This allows us to focus less on 'truth' and more on how and why patients' narratives are constructed in specific ways at specific times.

A number of methodological criteria informed the choice of approach and method (BNIM) in this study of motivation in mental health (Campbell-Breen, 2004). The first criterion was the ability of the methodology chosen to draw on life stories, thereby allowing meaning constructed through individual narrative about life and by incorporating relevant social, economic and environment factors (Gadamer, 1975). Secondly, the methodology sought to explore motivation from a range of experiences rather than just one specific experience or period in life (Alheit, 1994). Thirdly, the methodology offered access to the individual's own interpretive understanding and expression about actions and behaviours in life. The fourth criterion was the ability of the methodology to recognise that while individuals may or may not be able to articulate clear definitions about their own motivation (or any other research topic), their stories may provide a possible means to appreciate their motivation. The final criterion was that the chosen methodology should enable participants to choose what they want to talk about. After all, they are the experts in their own lives.

THE BIOGRAPHIC-NARRATIVE-INTERPRETIVE METHOD (BNIM)

While our general methodological framework helped us to approach the study of motivation, we still needed to develop methods of data collection and analysis that took account of these criteria. The highly structured, rigorous data collection and analysis procedures of the BNIM (Rosenthal, 1998) provided what we saw as an appropriate method, and also one that would enhance the trustworthiness and rigour of the research. While the recommended structure of interviewing and analysis below may appear prescriptive and rigid, procedures are in fact open, so that participants are encouraged to take control of what is spoken about.

Data are collected through three sequential subsets (stages) of questioning styles over two interviews. The first interview includes Subsets I and II. Subset I is characterised by a single, open, narrative-inducing question that aims to elicit the individual's 'whole life' story. Subset II is characterised by further narrative-inducing questions on topics raised earlier by the participant's story and in the sequence the participant has raised them. The second interview covers Subset III questions, which address apparent gaps in the story or where additional material relating to the research aims and first interview is sought. This incorporates both closed and open questioning styles. This collection procedure helps place the responsibility for constructing the narrative with the client, while limiting common therapeutic procedures of collecting data.

The process of analysis is distinguished by the separate involvement of the researcher and panels of independent individuals who are otherwise not involved in any other aspect of the research process. Both researcher and panel engage in a structured analysis procedure that addresses the separate components of the life story: the 'lived life' (biographical events in chronological order) and the 'told story' (the sequential narrative constructing the life). The researcher organises the transcripts of the interview by separating the data of the 'lived life' from those of the 'told story'. The panels develop hypotheses about motivation for each individual based on data presented separately from the 'lived life' and the 'told story'. These are then compared by the researcher in a final stage of analysis. The aim here is to develop insights about individual motivation from the whole life account, based on analysis of the component parts. The rationale for the data collection and analysis procedures is detailed below. (A more detailed account of the BNIM is provided by Wengraf, 2001.)

DOING THE RESEARCH

A CHALLENGE FROM CLINICIAN-GATEKEEPERS?

Researching the motivation of clients with mental health difficulties means gaining access to, and building relationships with people who are generally recognised to be vulnerable (Department of Health, 1999). The fact that we were researching mental health clients certainly affected the process through which we needed to negotiate access (Butler, 2003) and gain informed consent (Mazur, 2003). The clinician-gatekeepers played a role in influencing access and engagement during recruitment and interviewing.

We used clinicians in the recruitment process of clients because these were perceived to be vulnerable clients. We spent considerable time meeting clinical staff and explaining the research process to them. Two main difficulties became apparent. The first related to how gatekeepers viewed the issue of informed consent in relation to their clients. The second was the tendency of gatekeepers to select 'motivated' clients.

The first problem is illustrated by the following excerpt from Tanya's fieldnotes. This shows how gatekeepers gave precedence to clinical judgements about informed consent over clients' own ability or choice to give informed consent:

> I had received a signed, informed consent form from the client of a particular inpatient unit. I then contacted the staff in order to arrange a convenient time and place to see the client. I was told I could not see the client, and when I asked if it was because the client could not give informed consent, the reply was 'no, he can give consent, but the staff don't want him to see you'. [Fieldnotes: Contact with Gatekeeper in Unit 3]

Such responses suggest that clinical priorities and institutional power may influence the recruitment of vulnerable client groups into research (Thurgood, 2003).

The second problem, too, is evidenced by my fieldnotes. I found that gatekeepers were predetermining who was motivated and who was not, and that this may have restricted our access to particular types of accounts. Encounters with gatekeepers from two different units highlight the problem. In one unit, a gatekeeper told me:

> Oh, I know some really motivated patients that would enjoy doing this sort of thing.

In another unit I was told by a gatekeeper:

> I think some of my clients would be too disturbed to read the study information, so I won't even try and give it to them. [Fieldnotes: Contact with Gatekeeper in Unit 1]

While such views did pose a challenge, in the end we did not feel that they restricted our access to different client accounts. Our purposeful selection (Mason, 2002) sought to gain stories from clients using a range of mental health services and provide different types of accounts. We thereby hoped to gain access to a variety of life stories, presented in different ways. While some gatekeepers may have selected what they perceived to be 'motivated' clients, whether such clients would be perceived as motivated when analysed in the study was open to question. Time spent explaining the research methodology to clinicians and encouraging them to take it on board may have helped develop a relationship of trust and mutual respect between researcher and clinician. However, it did little to change this particular aspect of gatekeepers' behaviour.

DATA COLLECTION

In common with most users of this method, our initial question in Subset 1 was:

> Can you please tell me about the story of your life, all those events and experiences which were important for you. I will listen first. I won't interrupt. I'll take some notes so that I can ask you questions afterwards.

The purpose of this single narrative question is twofold. First, it aims to encourage participants to select and determine their own responses to a question relating to something in which they are expert: their life story. It also aims to limit the researcher's involvement in the initial stages of the interview procedure (Breckner, 1998) and to minimise the impact on the questioning process of the researcher's professional training biases.

Secondly, the single narrative question aims to give analytic importance to the way that topics are selected and spoken about by the participant (Rosenthal, 1998). It also makes it possible for subsequent analysis to identify notable omissions or differences in how the narrative is constructed at different points. As the participant talked in the Subset I stage of interviews, we took detailed notes on the topics and themes raised. This method of data collection places the client's meaning structures at the centre of the process, rather than locating them within the researcher's own predominant schema.

Once clients have completed their often lengthy story, Subset II interviewing begins. This is based on a review of the notes taken during Subset I. This stage of the interview is characterised by further 'narrative-inducing' questions (Chamberlayne and Spano, 2000). These are asked in the same sequence as the topics were originally raised by the participant. In Subset II, there is a continuing focus on the narrative the participant constructs. Participants are encouraged to expand on what they have already said, with the researcher resisting the temptation to introduce new topics.

The second interview (Subset III questions) is carried out once the initial analysis has been completed. By this stage, the researcher will have identified initial themes and narrative constructions. This enables apparent gaps and contradictions in a participant's life story to be addressed in the second interview. At this stage, too, the researcher is in a position to outline themes that may be relevant to a participant's motivation. Clarifying and checking this initial analysis with participants provides the basis for new questions, which may be either closed or open (Wengraf, 2001). However, even at this stage, a strong focus may remain on the data provided by the participant previously.

DATA ANALYSIS

The analysis process provides a structured, staged approach to the separate analysis of the 'lived life' and the 'told story'.

The first stage of the analysis is completed by the interviewer and enables the data to be prepared for presenting to the panel. The 'lived life' comprises those biographical events and actions that can in most cases be verified by some form of historical/official documentation: for example birth certificates, school and employment records and marriage certificates. As explained earlier, however, we did not attempt to verify the 'truthfulness' of the events in this study. Listening to the audiotapes enables the researcher to 'pull out' the participant's life events and arrange them chronologically, even if this involves altering the sequence in which they were presented in the interview. This process highlights the full temporality of life experience, while only emphasising actions.

The 'told story' addresses both the sequence of structural changes in the life story and the way events or actions are experienced (Wengraf, 2001). The researcher transcribes the interviews and presents the 'told story' in the same order that it is spoken about. The 'told story' therefore acknowledges where there is a change in speaker (from interviewer to interviewee and vice versa), a change in topic and a change in the way the narrative is presented (for example, a change from 'rich' description with causal links to a 'thin' listing of information). The structure of the story is important when interpreting meaning in narrative research (Rosenthal, 1993). The purpose of these early analysis stages is to present to the panel the component parts of the whole.

The process of analysing the 'lived life' (biographic data) and the 'told story' involves a group panel, composed of at least three members (facilitated by the researcher), who undertake datum-by-datum analysis of the 'parts' until all the data is presented from Subset I of the interview. The panel then builds predictive hypotheses in a process based partly on a grounded theory approach (Glaser and Strauss, 1967), and partly on developing counter-hypotheses in a form of emergent theorising (Mason, 2002). This process is continued until a structural hypothesis comes to be validated by data drawn from the whole interview (Chamberlayne and King, 1997).

Including panels in the research increases the range of experience and widens the perspectives brought to the hypothesising process. It therefore adds to what the researcher, who already is aware of the story as a whole, can bring to the process. This stage of analysis limits the possibility of the panel prematurely formulating hypotheses relating to motivation while remaining blind to the story as a whole. The use of panels thus enhances the hermeneutic circle of interpretation and strengthens the trustworthiness of the findings.

Data from the 'lived life' are presented in small data sets from the chronological life sequence (Breckner, 1998). In contrast, the 'told story' datum sets are characterised by changes in topics, speakers and the manner in which the story is told. Interpretation of data is done in sequence until all data is presented to the panel (Rosenthal, 2004). At each stage of the analysis process, the panel develops hypotheses about individual motivation in the 'lived life' and the 'told story' without knowledge of data from the other component part. The panel's analysis of the 'told story' involves developing a hypothesis for the client's system of knowledge, their interpretations of their life, and their classification of experiences into themes or ideas. This is done in order to highlight significant areas or gaps within the life story of which the client may be unaware (Rosenthal, 1993). Hypothesising about the 'told story' draws on the participant's own meaning structures. In the final stage the researcher compares the panel's hypotheses developed about motivation. The researcher's task now is to complete the part/whole process of hermeneutic interpretation. In the light of the interview (the whole) and the panel's interpretations of the 'lived life' and the 'told story' (the parts), the researcher seeks to develop a final appreciation of the client's motivation.

FINDINGS

This chapter uses the findings from the case of a single client, Paul (a pseudonym), to illustrate how BNIM helped us explore individual motivation. The text in small font is used to represent study fieldnotes, transcribed interviews and analysis records.

THE 'LIVED LIFE'

The panel analysis produced the following structural hypotheses relating to Paul's 'lived life':

Paul is the youngest of four boys. His brothers are fourteen, two and one (Josh) year older than Paul. [Researcher's summary of biographical data]

Early hypothesis building suggested to the panel that Paul seemed to have had no interaction with female role models throughout his life. He was seen to place importance on experiences involving his brothers, and specifically his youngest brother, Josh.

They had jobs at his father's hotel until their teenage years.

The importance of male role models and lack of female role models is further supported in the panel's hypothesis building on the basis of subsequent data. The relationship with his brother Josh is seen to continue as Paul gets older and begins his career:

Paul completes a mechanics apprenticeship, while Josh completes one in bricklaying. After finishing their apprenticeships, they travel around Europe together. When they return, Paul qualifies as a bricklayer and works with Josh in the UK and Germany.

The panel begins to develop hypotheses suggesting that Paul's many apparently successful life experiences demonstrate that he is a motivated individual who has been able to show initiative. Panel members were therefore surprised to encounter the following data:

> Paul and Josh return from Germany and a year later Paul has a 'horrendous nervous breakdown' [Transcript 1/31]. Tries and fails twice to complete a computer course. Relapsed once, and continues with outpatient therapy. **Unemployed since illness.**

The hypotheses the panel generates on the basis of this data conflict with those generated from earlier data. That Paul would become unwell had not been developed as a future possibility in the panel's earlier analysis. As the 'lived life' provides no insight into the individual's story surrounding the nervous breakdown, the panel is left uncertain about Paul's motivation. This indicates how insights gained from factual events may not be enough to appreciate an individual's motivation adequately.

THE 'TOLD STORY'

The themes raised by the panel in the hypothesis-building process of the 'told story' are similar to those gained in the 'lived life'. This similarity may be related to the way Paul presents the story. Although the story has an adequate chronology and can be followed as a sequence by the listener, it is told by Paul as if he were a detached observer of his own life. Paul does not give details of his own interpretation based on his past and present perspectives and experiences. He often presents his story in the formal language of a report. The only times when he gives some inkling of the feelings and emotions attached to particular experiences relate to instances spent with his brother. The panel's hypothesis suggests that male companionship and feelings of happiness can be most clearly linked to those times Paul spent with his brothers, in particular Josh. These, then, are construed as forming an important part of his meaning of motivation.

However, it must be noted that while the panel is able to develop some hypotheses about Paul's motivation from earlier life events, these appear to be in contradiction with the hypotheses built on the basis of Paul's later experiences. The hypotheses are therefore not fully supported by the data. This contradiction is exposed when Paul, going into a bit more detail about the circumstances of his illness, raises more questions than answers for this panel:

From training as a bricklayer, Paul jumps to telling the researcher about having a breakdown, which occurred about five years ago. He doesn't explain why he became ill, but rather relies on the explanations of the medical doctor, who says 'that's a horrendous breakdown . . . caused by stress and depression' [Transcript 1/31]. Paul talks about coming to OT, getting well and becoming unwell again, which he links to the fact that they have changed his medication. [Researcher summary of Paul's told story]

COMPARISON BETWEEN THE 'LIVED LIFE' AND THE 'TOLD STORY'

At the end of the analysis of Subset I, the researcher using BNIM will note any outstanding issues for the comparison of hypotheses from the 'lived life' and 'told story'. In the case of Paul, the panel remains unclear about the reasons for Paul becoming unwell. His story of his breakdown appears to conflict with previous hypothesis building by the panel. As analysis of Subset II continues, further insights into Paul's motivation emerge. The reasons behind his many career and adult life changes become more apparent. In particular, more is learnt about the importance of Josh in providing Paul with anchorage.

In response to the narrative-inducing questions asked in Subset II, Paul becomes more of a storyteller. He tells how he and Josh went travelling together:

> And ah, Josh was really good company, yeah. Um, yeah, that, that was the way we got round, just transport, trains. And it went on for about six or seven months. [Paul's Transcript 7/302–7/305]

That Josh, already working in Germany, convinced Paul to go out there and work for him seems to be an example of how Paul may be directed by his brother. It contradicts, or at least modifies, the hypothesis regarding Paul's 'initiative' developed by the panel from the 'lived life'. Paul also explains that on his return to the UK, Josh got him a job in the oil company where he was working as a manager.

At this stage in the interviewing process, Paul is asked for more information about the time he became ill. His account shows he has difficulty placing himself within that experience. He refers to 'authority' and uses the doctor's words rather than his own to explain what happened. His account of what happened immediately before and after his illness contains no references to Josh:

> Yeah um, (5) well the doctors don't really know why I became ill. Um, one day said it that was your depression starting up. The GP, told me 'well,

it's just one of them things that flairs up sort of thing'. So nobody can tell me what it is, but they just give me the tablets to treat it, sort of thing. So um, nothing really, I weren't doing nothing at the time to, start it up, it just happened. [Paul's Transcript 8/390–8/394]

In the light of the stories provided in Subset II, we hypothesise that Paul's motivation within his life is directed less by his own initiative than by his brother's.

In the second interview, this idea was probed further. When Paul is asked about his relationship with Josh, he responds:

Well, I definitely don't see him as much as I used to obviously 'cause he's married and things like that. But we're very friendly, maybe one argument ever. You know, we can trust each other. And, you know, we think a lot of each other, sort of thing. [Paul's Transcript 26/1275–1277]

When asked why he trained as a bricklayer, he says:

Yeah, well I at the time, all the brothers were never ever out of work and when I started as soon as I finished the training we had a really good session and everyone was, and since then it's been a struggle. [Paul's Transcript 26/1289–1291]

This statement conflicts with his earlier portrayal of his success stories in career and job roles, and suggests that Paul's reason is related to his relationship with Josh. The 'struggle' that Paul mentions appears to coincide with a time of less contact and direction from Josh – a time that began before the onset of Paul's illness. Paul seems unable at this point to 'see' himself within his own life story and appears not to recognise the part that Josh has played in his life and motivation.

Paul's case, and the hypothesis-building process around it, indicates how the use of BNIM reveals the contribution of life narratives to understanding meaning. In the course of the research, it became clear to us that only certain kinds of narrative allowed us as researchers, together with the panel, to appreciate an individual's meaning of motivation. Although Subset I had apparently provided enough information for the panel to generate workable hypotheses, this information did not prove sufficient. The panel was not able, on this basis, to generate structural hypotheses that could be supported by the data in Subset I. An analysis of Subsets II and III, taking into account the panel's analysis of Subset I, had to be completed before it was possible to construct a more robust final hypothesis about Paul's motivation in life.

REFLECTIONS

This review of how Paul's story was analysed using BNIM demonstrates that eliciting a comprehensive biographical history alongside storytelling can support an interpretation of his motivation, without having to seek some explicit formulation of motivation from him. However, to develop such an account requires the researcher to seek a particular type of constructed story, and takes on board clients' own interpretation of their lives. If we are to fully engage with clients' meanings, we need to make it possible for clients to tell stories that include not just events but also their own interpretation of events and experiences.

The rigorous approach to data collection and analysis provided by BNIM led us to attach importance to the meanings that individuals give to their own life events and experiences. In this study, such an approach supported a client-contextualised interpretation of motivation rather than one based on health professionals' judgements. By undertaking separate analyses of Paul's 'lived life' and 'told story', we were able to identify a particular relationship dynamic as central to an understanding and conceptualisation of Paul's motivation.

The findings produced by this provide evidence on which to question the adequacy of the frameworks used by health professionals in assessing and understanding motivation. Approaching motivation from a hermeneutic perspective encouraged us to view motivation within a context of individual life stories – a context broader than that constituted by illness or treatment.

One particular problem we encountered was how to present findings developed through multiple levels of analysis in a way that can be readily understood by readers. We sought to address this by presenting findings from various stages of the analysis, placing sections of the interview text alongside analysts' responses to these. By this means, the structured analysis procedure could be rendered more transparent to those encountering BNIM for the first time.

BNIM provides a rigorous approach to exploring the complexity of meaning. While such concepts as motivation may not be easy topics for interviewing purposes, the BNIM can provide insights that are firmly grounded in individuals' own accounts of their lives. In addition, by exploring it from a narrative, hermeneutic philosophy and in taking a BNIM approach, we have suggested that our meaning making about motivation may not be that of the clients if they were asked explicitly: 'What motivates you?' This is because we have argued that our approach to motivation allows meaning to be derived from the individuals' construction and interpretation of their life stories and not from what they say about motivation specifically. The motivational findings of this study therefore may not be something of which individuals are made consciously aware in their story constructions. Yet the BNIM provides a systematic approach to exploring differences in meanings derived from 'observed actions' and meanings derived from 'stories about actions'. Finally, by focusing on the construction of narrative, BNIM provides a rigorous way of appreciating mental health clients' stories that may not necessarily conform to expected narrative structures.

REFERENCES

Alheit, P. (1994) 'Everyday time and life time: On the problems of healing contradictory experiences of time', *Time and Society*, 3(3): 305–19.

Breckner, R. (1998) 'The biographic-interpretive method: Principles and procedures', in *SOSTRIS Working Paper 2: Case study materials: The early retired: Social strategies in risk societies*, London: University of East London.

Butler, J. (2003) 'Research in the place where you work: Some ethical issues', *Bulletin of Medical Ethics*, 185: 21–2.

Campbell-Breen, T. (2004) 'Motivation in mental health: A hermeneutic qualitative exploration of client and occupational therapist narratives', unpublished PhD thesis, Norwich: University of East Anglia.

Chamberlayne, P. and King, A. (1997) 'The biographical challenge of caring', *Sociology of Health and Illness*, 19(5): 601–21.

Chamberlayne, P. and Spano, A. (2000) 'Modernisation as lived experience: Contrasting case studies from the SOSTRIS project', in Chamberlayne, P., Bornat, J. and Wengraf, T. (eds), *The Turn to Biographical Methods in Social Science: Comparative Issues and Examples*, London: Routledge.

Denzin, N.K. (2000) 'Narrative's moment', in Andrews, M., Day Sclater, S., Squire, C. and Treacher, A. (eds), *Lines of Narrative: Psychosocial Perspectives*, London: Routledge.

Department of Health (1999) *National Service Framework for Mental Health: Modern Standards and Service Models*, London: Department of Health.

Gadamer, H.-G. (1975) *Truth and Method*, London: Sheed and Ward.

Glaser, B. and Strauss, A. (1967) *The Discovery of Grounded Theory: Strategies for Qualitative Research*, Chicago: Aldine de Gruyter.

Grondin, J. (2002) 'Gadamer's basic understanding of understanding', in Dostal, R.J. (ed.), *The Cambridge Companion to Gadamer*, Cambridge: Cambridge University Press.

Heidegger, M. (1967) *Being and Time* (trans. John Macquarrie and Edward Robinson), Oxford: Blackwell.

Maclean, N., Pound, P., Wolfe, C. and Rudd, A. (2000) 'Qualitative analysis of stroke patients' motivation for rehabilitation', *British Medical Journal*, 321: 1051–4.

Mason, J. (2002) *Qualitative Researching*, London: Sage Publications.

Mazur, D.J. (2003) 'Influence of the law on risk and informed consent', *British Medical Journal*, 327: 731–4.

Rosenthal, G. (1993) 'Reconstruction of life stories: Principles of selection in generating stories for narrative biographical interviews', in Josselson, R. and Lieblich, A. (eds), *The Narrative Study of Lives, Vol. 1*, Newbury Park, CA: Sage Publications.

Rosenthal, G. (1998) *The Holocaust in Three Generations: Families of Victims and Perpetrators of the Nazi Regime*, London: Cassell.

Rosenthal, G. (2004) 'Biographical research', in Seale, C., Gobo, G., Gubrium, J.F. and Silverman, D. (eds), *Qualitative Research Practice*, London: Sage Publications.

Sewards, T.V. and Sewards, M.A. (2003) 'Representations of motivational drives in mesial cortex, medial thalamus, hypothalamus and midbrain', *Brain Research Bulletin*, 61: 25–49.

Thurgood, G. (2003) 'I want a life story not a life sentence: Legal, ethical and human rights issues related to recording, transcribing and archiving oral history interviews', in Horrocks, C., Kelly, N., Roberts, B. and Robinson, D. (eds), *Narrative, Memory and Health*, Huddersfield: University of Huddersfield Press.

Wengraf, T. (2001) *Qualitative Research Interviewing: Biographic Narrative and Semi-Structured Methods*, London: Sage Publications.

Wong, A.H.C. and Van Tol, H.H.M. (2003) 'Schizophrenia: From phenomenology to neurobiology', *Neuroscience and Biobehavioural Reviews*, 27: 269–306.

12

Empowering Young People through Participatory Research?

ANNE KILLETT

What happens when children and young people are referred to mental health services? Do they get the help they want or expect? What sense do they make of their experiences? As an occupational therapist working in child and adolescent mental health services (CAMHS), I had the opportunity to pursue these questions while studying part-time for a Doctorate in Education (EdD). At that time the service was under pressure to reduce waiting lists. This meant that difficult decisions were being taken about whom the service would be offered to, and which interventions resources should be put into. One viewpoint was noticeably absent from the discussion, with its focus on costs, benefits, resources and evidence. The group of people whose needs were being discussed and planned for seemed to have no say at all in the process.

Yet I knew that young people did make observations about the interventions they were offered, and did have views about things they found helpful or less helpful. If and when we clinicians were ready to listen to them, young people wanted to negotiate such issues as which clinicians they saw, what was discussed, who went to sessions with them and how often they were seen. The problem was how to represent young people's views in the public arena so that they became

Qualitative Research for Allied Health Professionals: Challenging Choices. Edited by Linda Finlay and Claire Ballinger.   Copyright 2006 by John Wiley & Sons Ltd.   ISBN 0-470-01963-8.

'admissible evidence'. Tackling this challenge became the focus of my research.

My aim was to find out about young people's experiences in a way that valued and respected the young people themselves. Children and young people typically do not have much control or authority over those parts of their lives that are bound up with institutions (such as education or health services). Where a young person's mental health comes into question, even the limited control the young person has may evaporate completely. It was all too easy, I felt, for such a scenario to be played out in the research process. My first challenge, then, was to find an appropriate methodology.

METHODOLOGY: IN SEARCH OF A RESPECTFUL RELATIONSHIP

Studies of mental health services for children and adolescents are interesting on two counts: the questions they have tackled and the ways they have involved young people in the research. Research in this area could be grouped into four broad themes. These include research into the technology of interventions, including in the areas of psychopharmacology, neurochemistry and psychological interventions; 'client satisfaction'; research into the experiences and views of young service users; and evaluations of interventions (e.g. Fonagy et al., 2002). While it could be seen as respectful to consider users' views of satisfaction with services, the very nature and scope of services offered stem from the relationship between funding priorities nationally and locally, and notions of what there is evidence for. Services have had little influence on which topics are explored to develop evidence.

In general, young people who use mental health services have had little influence on which topics are explored to develop evidence. Research has typically defined young people in terms of their symptoms: for example as 'maltreated youth' (Garland et al., 2000, p. 130), as 'mixed neurotic and conduct disordered' (Pyne et al., 1986, p. 66), as 'high-risk adolescents' (Ungar and Teram, 2000, p. 233) or even as 'adolescent self-poisoners' (Burgess et al., 1998, p. 210). Such language speaks of a gulf between the writers and those who are being written about. It is hard to imagine young people choosing such words to describe themselves. If this is the language of the evidence that informs practitioners, it seems to reduce the possibility of effective communication between practitioners and service users. The two groups seem destined to remained locked in their separate worlds. The words we use to talk and think are fundamental to our understanding. We need to pay attention both to how we describe people and to how we communicate with them. As Reason (1994) notes:

> we can only truly do research *with* persons if we engage with them *as* persons, as co-subjects and thus as co-researchers: hence co-operative inquiry, participatory research, research partnerships. (Reason, 1994, p. 10, emphasis in original)

Reading Reason's book was what first aroused my interest in participative research. Participative research has a long history in community development (Swantz, 1996; Hall, 2001). Hall (2001) characterises such research as a three-stranded enterprise combining social investigation, education and action. Those who have used the approach have usually done so with the aim of producing knowledge and actions useful to the community involved. In this respect the approach has much in common with action research (Reason and Bradbury, 2001). However, participatory research also aims to build participants' awareness, to boost their confidence in their own knowledge and experience (Reason, 1994). Participatory approaches are increasingly in evidence in health care settings, both among service providers and among service users (Ramon *et al.*, 2001; Burke *et al.*, 2003).

In participatory research the community affected by the research (for example a group of people using a service or a team of people working together) is involved in the research at as early a stage as possible. These people are seen as experts in the particular situation and their involvement in developing the questions to be explored is therefore essential. They may develop the methods for the research and go on to gather the data, or may commission others to do so (Rose, 1999; Ochoka *et al.*, 2002). The methods (as distinct from the methodology) that might be used could involve qualitative or quantitative methods of gathering and analysing data. The important distinguishing feature of participatory research is its methodology. This insists that participants are involved in the key decisions about the research.

Decisions about such issues as the questions to be investigated or the meanings that can be made from the data have profound implications for any group of people who are subject to research. Oliver (1992) argues that, far from being 'neutral', the words and terms used in questions indicate the categories in which the researcher aims to place participants. They indicate the researcher's views about the nature and likely causality of the issues being explored. By way of example, Oliver cites questions from a survey of disabled adults conducted by the Office of Population Censuses and Surveys: 'Can you tell me what is wrong with you?' and 'What complaint causes your difficulty in holding, gripping or turning things?'

Against these, Oliver suggests the following alternatives: 'What is wrong with society?' and 'What defects in the design of everyday equipment like jars, bottles and tins cause you difficulty in holding, gripping or turning them?' (Oliver, 1992, p. 104)

Swantz, a major proponent of participatory approaches in research, also argues that research is not a neutral activity. For Swantz, it is unavoidably political (Swantz, 1988). As she points out, 'In view of the fact that a mode of analysis may contribute to further subjection, of people in general and of women, the theoretical approach is crucial' (Swantz, 1985, p. 3).

Participatory research aims to involve research participants in these decisions. At the same time, it concedes that issues about the relative power held by different players need to be explicitly examined. For example, a person coming into a situation with professional or academic qualifications may well be seen by people without such qualifications as an expert whose opinions should carry more weight.

Critics of participatory research argue that, despite their emancipatory aspirations, researchers using this approach have frequently ignored power issues within the research process. Healey (2001) points to studies that have not acknowledged the powerful position of professional researchers working as facilitators of participatory research with groups of people. Cleaver (1999) highlights power differences within communities engaged in participatory research.

In the case of my own research, I was concerned that young people who used mental health services had little or no voice in decisions about who would be offered the services and what exactly would be offered. The evidence used to inform such decisions seemed to me to pigeon-hole young people as 'research subjects'. Once they were placed in this slot, only those aspects of the young people that were believed to be 'relevant' to the researcher's agenda were considered. Yet at the same time government rhetoric was exhorting researchers to involve users in service evaluation and development (e.g. Department of Health, 2002). I thought that a participative approach to the question that was interesting me would not only produce useful information, but would also help empower the young people who got involved.

DOING THE RESEARCH: THE CHALLENGE TO BE CONSISTENT WITH PRINCIPLES

Having decided to use a participative approach, I sought a way of sharing the research process with the young participants from as early a stage as possible. This was to enable the people actually using the service to shape the areas to be explored. To be consistent with the aim of partnership with participants, I had to think about the influence I wielded, even at the point of recruiting people as participants. My plan was to invite young people to meet in a group to explore ideas about the process of doing the research. I was keeping an open mind about what methods any participants might develop. Young people might well have more relevant ideas than me about how they or their peers could best reveal their experiences. They might, for example, want to use pictures, photographs, perhaps even video. If I was to involve young people actively in this project, I needed to get their involvement all the way through. This included involving them in the analysis of data and the presentation of findings.

NEGOTIATING WITH OTHER PLAYERS

I sought to recruit young people who were currently using, or who had recently used, the CAMH service in which I was working. As I thought about how soon I could try to involve young people in the process, I confronted my first challenge. I could not begin to talk to people who were patients about my research until I had ethical approval. As I prepared to seek approval from the local research ethics committee, the contrast between the participatory philosophy I was aspiring to and the paternalism of the health service was immediately highlighted. The application form for ethical approval that I completed had to be approved and signed by a medical director.

There was no support for my initial idea of developing a 'users' group' alongside my research project. Concern was expressed that such a group would be formed of the 'wrong' people, people with an 'axe to grind'. The literature on user involvement in mental health services (e.g. Rogers *et al.*, 1993) reveals this to be a familiar argument: one of several used to undermine the views of service users, especially where such views are critical of mental health services. In some cases, the validity of users' views will be questioned on methodological grounds. It will be argued that because these people held particular opinions they were obviously biased and do not represent the majority view. Views may be dismissed on the grounds of irrationality; they may be said to be part and parcel of the service user's 'symptoms'. Patients' views will be given less credence than those of carers or relatives where these views differ. Alternatively, views may be accepted, at least in part, where they happen to coincide with the professionals' own views (Rogers *et al.*, 1993). Certain groups may simply not be present in the research process at all: professionals may claim that their diagnosis means they lack the capability of making informed decisions about giving their consent.

Yet, as personal accounts testify, people who have experienced mental health services are well able to both describe and analyse their experiences of those services (see for example Read and Reynolds, 1996; Pegler, 2004).

I was pleased, however, that the committee accepted the case I made in my proposal, especially bearing in mind that I was asking for approval to conduct research with people who could be considered as additionally vulnerable because of their young age and their involvement with mental health services. There were two aspects of my proposal that I thought might cause particular concern. The first was that it would not be consistent to state exactly what questions would be addressed and what methods used. In participatory research, as I have explained, the distinguishing feature of the methodology is that the participants develop the questions and are centrally involved in determining methods.

The second aspect I feared might be controversial was my position towards informing my participants' general practitioners (GPs) about their patients' involvement in my research. The form asked for a justification if this was not to happen. The underlying assumption seemed to be that there ought to be a direct relationship between GP and researcher. My position on this was rather different. While I recognised that such a relationship might be necessary on safety grounds in the case of pharmacological trials or where interventions by GPs and by researchers might interact or overlap, I argued that even in these instances the patient should be involved in any discussions or information loops between the researcher and the GP. For the specific research that I was proposing, I argued that any decision to inform GPs that their patients were taking part in the research should remain with the participants. Confidentiality is an important and sensitive issue for young people involved with mental health services. I argued that I would not be able to give participants any justification for informing their GP that they were taking part. If placed under any obligation to inform GPs, I would then have to negotiate with participants what information would or would not be disclosed to GPs. This, I argued, would add another layer to the complexity of participants giving their informed consent.

I was pleased to find that the ethics committee accepted these points. The committee was perhaps reassured by the rigour of my approach to recruiting people to take part in the research. When they asked for greater clarification about how any data would be analysed, I pointed out that I needed to remain open about this, given my starting point of being open about the methods that might be used. I could not be categorical about how data would be analysed because I did not know what form the data might be in. What I was able to say was that I aimed to involve participants in the data analysis process.

The next stage was to negotiate my research plans with the rest of the CAMHS team. This negotiation was important, as people working in the service could feel very vulnerable as a result of young people talking about their experiences of the service. As with the issue of involving GPs, the question at the centre of the negotiation was whether I should directly inform team members of their patients' involvement in my research. In the information sheet I had prepared I said that I would not inform any clinician (that is, any person from the multidisciplinary CAMHS team) about the involvement of their young patients in my research. If a young person wanted to tell their clinician, or talk to them about taking part, that was fine; the decision was theirs. Equally, I was clear that I would not look at participants' medical records. If I had prior knowledge about them I would aim not to bring this into the research. I could have prior knowledge if a young person who I had worked with opted to take part in the research. I could also have prior knowledge if I had been part of a team discussion about a young person whom another clinician had seen. These considerations were very important: they ensured that during the research participants kept control of information about themselves.

RECRUITING PARTICIPANTS

As I entered the recruitment phase, I was clear that I could not switch in and out of my power-sharing mode. My position as an adult, a therapist and a researcher endowed me with power. How, then, to square this with the ethical consideration that people taking part in research do so only on the basis of freely given informed consent (Masson, 2000,

p. 40)? As Masson points out, children and young people may fear that they will be penalised for not taking part if someone in a powerful relationship with them approaches them. How could I avoid using my influence when recruiting would-be participants?

I decided that advertising offered a way round this problem. Here I adopted the simplest form: the display of posters. The local research ethics committee, which asked to see the posters I was planning to use, advised that it should be made clear that responding to the poster did not 'imply any degree of commitment' and that if people responded to the advertisement but then decided not to participate, any record of their name would be destroyed.

By using posters, I was asking people to 'opt in' if they wanted to take part in the research. I displayed the posters in the waiting rooms of the two CAMHS involved in the study. I also negotiated with a social services base that supported young people living independently, a non-statutory youth advice project and the local authority youth service, asking them to display posters and flyers that young people could take away. By publicising the research in these additional locations, I hoped to get the views of young people who might have been offered the service but had not taken it up, or who had wanted help from the service but had not been able to get referred to it. I emphasised to the staff at these different locations, and also to my colleagues, that I wasn't asking them to recruit people to the project, or even to raise the subject with young people. I did, however, want them to be helpful to any young people who approached them for more information, or who wanted to talk about taking part. I made a point of discussing the project and its ethos with people in each organisation.

I was aware that it was asking a lot of a young person in a waiting room, who was perhaps feeling anxious or concerned about coming to a service, to attend to a poster, take the active step of filling in a reply slip and then hand it to reception staff or put it in the post. In terms of research conventions, there is an unavoidable bias in recruiting in this way. This method is biased in favour of people with a functional level of literacy. It is likely to attract people with a certain amount of self-confidence. It might be argued that people with 'extreme' experiences, whether positive or negative, would be more likely to respond. This did not seem to be the case in my own research, where young people who mentioned their reasons for getting involved described wanting to take part in some activity or to meet other young people. In any case, discussion of 'sample bias' is not seen as relevant by adherents of participative research. Here, those taking part in research are not seen as 'representative' of any particular group or category. Instead, participants are viewed as experts in their own experience (Heron, 1996).

THE RESPONSE: NEGOTIATIONS

Once the posters were up, I waited anxiously, aware that it was asking a lot for people to volunteer. Would there be a flood of interested enquiries? Or would I hear nothing? Six months down the line, would I be caught up in my research or would I be involved in a drastic rethink?

The response was somewhere in the middle. About 16 young people responded to the posters by leaving their contact details with the receptionists and asking for more information. I discussed with them their level of participation and gave them information sheets and consent forms. Those who were 16 or over were able to give their own consent to take part in the research. However, those under the age of 16 needed their parent or guardian to consent on their behalf (see Masson, 2000, for further discussion of this issue). In the end nine participants were involved the project.

The next challenge was to deal with responses from the participants, which came over a period of months. There seemed to be a need to bring participants together as a group. Aware that I could easily be seen as an authority figure, I tried to make all arrangements for group meetings on the basis of negotiation. I learnt so much from this process. For example, I came face to face with the high levels of responsibility some of the participants shouldered: some had part-time jobs or family childcare responsibilities. I learnt that some were managing the complexities of maintaining relationships with parents who no longer lived with the family. In such cases, a young person would need to check arrangements for coming to the group meeting with two parents living in two different places. The participants had differing views on where to meet. While one suggested meeting in a café, another said they would feel too anxious to do so and preferred to meet at the CAMH centre. Much of this negotiation was carried on over the phone. While I was open with parents about who I was and why I was ringing, I was firm about negotiating directly with the young people themselves. Parents to whom I spoke in the course of these phone calls seemed to concur with this approach; none tried to make or stop arrangements on behalf of their son or daughter.

Despite all the careful negotiations, only one person out of five came to the group meeting. At this point I had a handful of people who had given their consent to take part in the research. Three of these had told me, during the course of a discussion, that they wanted to take part as researchers in addition to contributing data about their experiences. Two then regularly came in search of me whenever they had appointments at the service. They were eager to know when they would be able to do something. In effect, I was conducting my research with individual participants rather than with a group. To what extent did this matter? My emphasis was still on negotiation, rather than on 'instructing' my participants. But working with individuals rather than a group did make a difference. Encouraging an individual to become actively involved in generating questions and methods would place heavy demands on that individual's time and energy. It was also difficult for me to 'water down' my influence where the interaction was between myself and only one other. Had I been able to negotiate the forming of a group of participants, this might have provided a context in which peer support could have flourished. It might, too, have provoked more ideas about the research, including challenges to my own thoughts and observations.

Eventually, constrained by a time limit imposed by my decision to leave my job, I decided I had to take the project forward with the individuals who were keen to be involved. I therefore offered to talk with these people about their experiences. I was disappointed that I was not fulfilling my commitment to a participatory approach. Instead, I acted as an individual researcher involved in asking individual young people about their experiences, recording conversations and transcribing their accounts. This felt like a major compromise. At the same time, all of these young people had volunteered: clearly they wanted to take part in something.

The fact that two participants agreed to contribute to the analysis of the data maintained a participative element at the crucial stage of making meaning. This participative element was, however, constrained by several factors. For a start, there was a limit to how much time it seemed reasonable to ask of the young people involved. In addition, I did not have participants' explicit consent to show their interview transcripts to other participants. I therefore constructed themed abstracts from selected, anonymised pieces of data. Again, I was painfully aware of my power to select what I saw as the principal themes emerging from the data. In some cases, however, the young people who helped with the analysis (each of whom I met individually) did see things in the data that I didn't see.

FINDINGS

The young participants in the research emphasised the importance of the relationship they were offered by the clinicians they saw. They found it helpful when they felt they were seen as 'human beings' who had other sides to them, and were not just seen in terms of problems. Where clinicians offered them time and friendliness this was highly valued. However, three participants also said that at times it was important for the clinician to put some pressure on the young person to speak about difficult issues.

The participants showed that they had thought about the meaning of diagnostic labels such as depression and attention deficit disorder. Their responses to such labels were not simplistic. At least one participant rejected a label they had been given. Like adults engaged in service provision and development, these young people theorised about the causes of their difficulties. To what extent, they wondered, did people inherit things from their parents? How much were people affected by things that happened to them? Some expressed frustration over their inability to influence the type of intervention they were offered. In one case, for example, a young person had only been offered medication where they felt they needed practical advice and help to deal with anger. Others said that they wanted more help with family issues.

REFLECTIONS

My aim at the outset had been to facilitate far more participation than I managed. I found it difficult to use this approach as there was no pre-existing group or community. Young people attending individual or family appointments at outpatient services do not constitute a group or community, and might not want to give themselves the identity of belonging to such a group or community. However, adopting a participatory approach to research did offer dividends. For one thing, I placed emphasis on developing relationships with the participants that were respectful of their knowledge and experience. This had effects throughout the research process. It made me consider in detail how I could invite people to take part, being aware of the potential pressures my position could bring to bear on them. It put me in the position of respecting what they had to say, of accepting their comments as valid rather than simply as evidence for my theory building. It set the stage for a more even-handed dialogue. One thing to emerge from our conversations was the degree to which young mental health service users engage in the same debates as the adults organising and providing those services. This came to the fore particularly at the stage when the analysis of data was shared with participants. The research underlined the point that young people, far from being passive recipients of services, are active players who theorise about the nature and causality of mental health and illness, and critically evaluate the treatment they receive.

My starting point in this research was to respect the knowledge and experience of the people who might take part, rather than to see participants simply as sources of data. What I learnt in the process of the research was that however participatory an approach I devised, I would not be in a position to empower my participants. As Freire (1973) has pointed out, people cannot be empowered by others; they can only empower themselves. Where I can make a contribution is to influence the climate of service delivery, to encourage it to be one in which young people are listened to and communicated with respectfully. I need to empower myself to argue the case that service providers at all levels should find ways to join in the questioning and theorising in which young people are already engaged. Perhaps then collaborative service development, with young people's needs to the fore, can become the norm.

REFERENCES

Burgess, S., Hawton, K. and Loveday, G. (1998) 'Adolescents who take overdoses: Outcomes in terms of changes in psychopathology and the adolescents' attitudes to care and to their overdose', *Journal of Adolescence*, 21: 209–18.

Burke, A., McMillan, J., Cummins, L., Thompson, A., Forsyth, W., McLellan, J., Snow, L., Fraser, A., Fraser, M., Fulton, C., McGrindle, E., Gillies, L., LeFort, S., Miller, G., Whitehall, J., Wilson, J., Smith, J. and Wright, D. (2003) 'Setting up participatory research: A discussion of the initial stages', *British Journal of Learning Disabilities*, 31: 65–9.

Cleaver, F. (1999) 'Paradoxes of participation: Questioning participatory approaches to development', *Journal of International Development*, 11: 597–612.

Department of Health (2002) *Involving Patients and the Public in Health Care*, London: HMSO.

Fonagy, P., Target, M., Cottrell, D., Phillips, J. and Kurtz, Z. (2002) *What works for whom? A Critical Review of Treatments for Children and Adolescents*, New York: Guildford.

Freire, P. (1973) *Education: The Practice of Freedom*, London: Writers and Readers Publishing Cooperative.

Garland, A., Saltzman, M. and Aarons, G. (2000) 'Adolescent satisfaction with mental health services: Development of a multidimensional scale', *Evaluation and Program Planning*, 23(2, May): 165–75.

Hall, B. (2001) 'I wish this were a poem of practices of participatory research', in Reason, P. and Bradbury, H. (eds), *Handbook of Action Research, Participative Inquiry and Practice*, London: Sage Publications.

Healey, K. (2001) 'Participatory action research and social work: A critical appraisal', *International Social Work*, 44 (1): 93–105.

Heron, J. (1996) *Co-operative Inquiry: Research into the Human Condition*, London: Sage Publications.

Masson, J. (2000) 'Researching children's perspectives: Legal issues', in Lewis, A. and Lindsay, G. (eds), *Researching Children's Perspectives*, Buckingham: Open University Press.

Ochoka, J., Janzen, R. and Nelson, G. (2002) 'Sharing power and knowledge: Professional and mental health consumer/survivor researchers working together in a participatory action research project', *Psychiatric Rehabilitation Journal*, 25(4): 379–87.

Oliver, M. (1992) 'Changing the social relations of research production?', *Disability, Handicap and Society*, 7(2): 101–14.

Pegler, J. (2004) *A Can of Madness*, London: Chipmunkapublishing.

Pyne, N., Morrison R. and Ainsworth, P. (1986) 'A consumer survey of an adolescent unit', *Journal of Adolescence*, 9: 63–72.

Ramon, S., Castillo, H. and Morant, N. (2001) 'Experiencing personality disorder, a participative research', *International Journal of Social Psychiatry*, 47(4): 1–15.

Read, J. and Reynolds J. (1996) *Speaking Our Minds: An Anthology of Personal Experiences of Mental Distress and its Consequences*, Buckingham: Open University.

Reason, P. (ed.) (1994) *Participation in Human Inquiry*, London: Sage Publications.

Reason, P. and Bradbury, H. (eds) (2001) *Handbook of Action Research, Participative Inquiry and Practice*, London: Sage Publications.

Rogers, A., Pilgrim, D. and Lacey, R. (1993) *Experiencing Psychiatry: Users' Views of Services*, Basingstoke: Macmillan.

Rose, D. (1999) 'Do it yourselves', *Mental Health Care*, 2(5): 174–7.

Swantz, M.-L. (1985) *Women in Development: A Creative Role Denied? The Case of Tanzania*, London: C. Hurst and Co.

Swantz, M.-L. (1988) 'Participatory inquiry as an instrument of grass-roots development', in Reason, P. (ed.), *Human Inquiry in Action: Developments in New Paradigm Research*, London: Sage Publications, pp. 127–43.

Swantz, M.-L. (1996) 'A personal position paper on participatory research: Personal quest for living knowledge', *Qualitative Inquiry*, 2(1): 120–36.

Ungar, M. and Teram, E. (2000) 'Drifting toward mental health, high risk adolescents and the process of empowerment', *Youth and Society*, 32(2): 228–52.

13

The Embodied Experience of Multiple Sclerosis: An Existential-Phenomenological Analysis

LINDA FINLAY

A number of qualitative research studies have shown the potentially devastating impact that chronic illnesses such as multiple sclerosis can have on individuals' lives. This impact has been characterised as 'biographical disruption' (Bury, 1982) and 'narrative wreckage' (Frank, 1995).

In the case of multiple sclerosis (MS), Toombs writes that 'To live with multiple sclerosis is to experience a global sense of disorder – a disorder which incorporates a changed relation with one's body, a transformation in the surrounding world, a threat to the self, and a change in one's relation to others' (1995, p. 12). Koopman and Schweitzer (1999) pick up these themes, showing how the trauma of the body's 'betrayal' leads individuals to embark on a personal journey that, though potentially transformative, is essentially lonely, confusing and challenging.

It is important to recognise that multiple sclerosis is an extraordinarily variable disease – both in how the 'bewildering array' of symptoms manifest and in the course and prognosis of the condition (Toombs, 1995). Every person with multiple sclerosis has a different story to tell. For this reason, I embarked on some case-study research

Qualitative Research for Allied Health Professionals: Challenging Choices. Edited by Linda Finlay and Claire Ballinger.   Copyright 2006 by John Wiley & Sons Ltd.   ISBN 0-470-01963-8.

that involved approaching several individuals with multiple sclerosis. I wanted to hear – and honour – each of their special stories. This chapter seeks to tell one of the stories I heard: the story of Ann and her lived experience of having multiple sclerosis.

The chapter starts by outlining the key ideas underpinning **existential-phenomenological** methodology. I then describe how I applied this method in practice, sharing some of the challenges I faced. (As an experienced phenomenological researcher, my challenges were less about the choices I was making and more about how to do the phenomenology well enough to do justice to Ann's story.) Next, I outline those findings that specifically relate to the themes of 'embodiment' and 'sociality' (relations with others). I give these findings some emphasis in order to demonstrate what I see as the potential of phenomenological analyses to probe experience in depth and with some poetry. In the final reflection section, I evaluate the study and consider the role Ann played in our collaboration. Specifically, I reject the notion of 'participant validation' in favour of collaboration done in a spirit of openness and sharing.

METHODOLOGY: EXISTENTIAL PHENOMENOLOGY

> All my knowledge of the world . . . is gained from . . . experience of the world . . . To return to things themselves is to return to that world which precedes knowledge. (Merleau-Ponty, 1962, pp. viii–ix)

Phenomenology is concerned with the way things appear to people. 'It is the interrogation of the phenomenon in its appearing which allows us to recognise, to verbalise, maybe for the first time, the taken-for-granted which always lay right there, unrecognised . . . as part of the phenomenon' (Ashworth, 2003, p. 146). Resisting any rush to explanation, it stays as far as possible with descriptions of the person's experience. This commitment to description is revealed in two stages. First, the individual participant provides a 'naïve' (natural) description of a specific experience or situation. Then the researcher seeks, through their own descriptive efforts, to capture and explicate that experience.

The phenomenological movement was initiated by Husserl (1970) as a radically new way of doing philosophy. Later theorists, such as Heidegger (1962), have recast the phenomenological project, moving away from a philosophical discipline that focuses on consciousness and essences of phenomena towards elaborating existential and hermeneutic (interpretive) dimensions.

Existential phenomenologists are concerned with those issues that all humans confront to do with life and death. As humans, all of us question who we are and the meaningfulness of our lives. We are aware of the flow of time and our finiteness: we know we cannot last for ever. Along with our capacity to be reflexive (self-aware), we have an awareness of our own agency and our ability to do, to act purposefully. We are faced with myriad choices about how to *be*, both in our present relationships and in the future.

Existential phenomenologists focus on all these 'universal horizons' of experience. Specifically, they examine the life world (*Lebenswelt*) to do with being a body in space; being a self in time; and living with others. The term 'life world' directs attention to the individual's lived situation and social world rather than to some inner world of introspection.

Whichever variant of phenomenology is adopted, the aim for research is the same: to describe the everyday world as we immediately experience it. Importantly, this world is pre-reflective – it takes place before we think about it or put it into language.

Phenomenology asks: 'What is this kind of experience like?' The first challenge for phenomenological researchers like myself is to help participants express their sense of self/embodiment and lived relations with others as directly as possible. We then have to find a way to express this in language, a way that captures the complexity, ambiguities and nuances of the experience described.

The phenomenological method (Giorgi, 1985; Valle and Halling, 1989) is posited on the ongoing effort of the researcher to suspend or 'bracket' previous assumptions or understandings. Critics often misunderstand this to mean that an effort is being made to be 'objective' and unbiased. In fact, existential phenomenologists take the position that there is no such thing as presupposition-free knowledge; they argue that all description is already interpretation. In the 'bracketing' process, the researcher is attempting to see the world differently and to attend more actively to the participant's own way of seeing the world. The researcher strives for an open 'phenomenological attitude': they seek to be open to the Other, to put aside (to the extent possible) their own as well as more general cultural understandings of the world.

Using a range of research methods, including interviews and personal diary accounts, phenomenologists ask participants to describe their experience by posing such questions as: 'Could you describe a typical day?' or 'Can you describe that particular incident in more detail?' To analyse how participants respond to such questions, researchers begin by immersing themselves in what the participant has said or written. Their aim is thereby to empathise with the participant's situation and tune in to existential dimensions of that situation. For instance, researchers might pose the question: 'How is this person experiencing their day?' They might then seek to apply such notions as 'felt space' and 'felt time'. For example, what is the participant's experience in terms of felt space? Do they feel safe, free, trapped, exposed, small . . . ? In terms of felt time, does the participant seem to be experiencing this as pressured, slow, discontinuous . . . ?

The person's sense of past, present and future constitutes the horizons of their temporal landscape. The researcher aims to transpose themselves empathically and imaginally into the Other (Finlay, 2005). Rogers offers a benchmark definition of this process:

> It means entering the private world of the other and becoming thoroughly at home in it. It involves being sensitive, moment to moment, to the changing felt meanings which flow in this other person . . . It means temporarily living in his/her life, moving about in it delicately without making judgements . . . as you look with fresh and unfrightened eyes . . . (Rogers, 1975, p. 3)

The analysis then moves into the writing phase. Here phenomenologists try to bring the specific lived experience alive, to capture it through narrative or in terms of themes. Through the process of writing and rewriting, the researcher aims to go ever deeper, to identify multiple layers of meaning and lay bare certain truths while retaining the ambiguity and fragility of experience. In this respect, phenomenological research is somewhat akin to the writing of poetry. As Van Manen puts it, such research involves an 'untiring effort to author a sensitive grasp of being itself' (Van Manen, 1990, p. 132).

DOING THE RESEARCH

In the research example described for this chapter, I adopted a case-study method. This approach provided a first-person account that I analysed using an existential-phenomenological method. The idiographic approach adopted makes no assumption of an intersubjectively shared reality common to different individuals suffering from the same diagnosis. In other words, the focus was on the individual experience of Ann, my participant. I needed to keep reminding myself that Ann's story might or might not mirror the experience of others who have multiple sclerosis.

Throughout both the interview and the analysis, I attempted to set aside my previous assumptions and understandings. I strove to adopt an open presence to Ann's story as it unfolded; I sought to perceive in a new and different way. Along with every other phenomenologist, I struggled in the process. Sometimes I was less than successful. As an occupational therapist I have some familiarity with the clinical features of multiple sclerosis. Occasionally, seeing Ann through my 'therapist eyes', I found myself regarding her neurological problems as relatively 'mild'. At these times I didn't listen carefully enough to her story. I caught myself feeling that 'I'd heard such stories many times before'. In my more successful bracketing moments, I realised I had almost missed hearing how her life had been derailed. I understood that I needed to leave my own perspective aside in order to tune into Ann's priorities: for instance, her experience of feeling unable to caress, and so express her love for, her children.

I interviewed Ann on two occasions, using an in-depth, relatively nondirective approach. In the first interview Ann told her story. In the second, I started by laying out some of the themes by which I had been struck from the previous interview. Ann then responded to these, where necessary, elaborating on what she had said earlier to help me to understand her perspective better. I strove to be an interested, nonjudgemental listener and to promote natural, spontaneous conversation. I accepted Ann's expressions, both in the sense of not judging them and in the sense of assuming that they reflected her perceptions of her life world. Here I was on more familiar and comfortable ground. As a therapist I felt well practised in interviewing someone about their experiences, feelings and daily struggles.

After the interviews, I sought a way to analyse the data – a labour-intensive stage of the project. I had always loved the work of Wertz (1983) and found the analytical steps he outlined helpful (see Finlay, 1999, for a précis of this work). Wertz recommends taking repeated, systematic readings of the transcript towards exploring recurrent existential themes. I focused on seven existential dimensions of the life world: Ann's sense of embodiment; selfhood; sociality; temporality; spatiality; project; and discourse. These interlinked 'fractions' (Ashworth, 2003) acted as a lens through which to view the data. I found it helpful to focus on one dimension at a time. When focusing on embodiment, for example, I would ask: 'What is Ann's subjective sense of her body? How does she experience and move in her body? Does she feel big, small, clumsy, happy, tense, comfortable, disconnected, in pain?'

My next step was to capture in writing what I saw as the emergent themes. The challenge here was to express the ambiguity, ambivalence and messiness of Ann's experience. This proved far from easy. I would laboriously fill page after page on just one idea, perhaps elaborating a particular metaphor that had come to mind. I sometimes worried about this. Might I not be simply indulging myself, taking off on a flight of literary fancy? Was I still writing about Ann? To help me stay anchored and focused on the empirical project, I tried as much as I could to focus in on Ann's actual words and work them into the emerging text.

The final stage of the analysis saw me pulling Ann's story together to form a narrative. Here, I condensed the descriptive material I had gathered into what seemed to be key existential themes. This writing stage confronted me with a new challenge. I am a therapist and academic, not a writer. Could I do justice to Ann's life world? Could I do justice to phenomenology? Why had I chosen a method that is so time consuming and so demanding in terms of literary skill?

FINDINGS

With a successful marriage, two lovely children (a boy aged 8 and a girl aged 3) and a job she enjoyed, Ann was happy. Then one day, numbness in the finger tips of her right (dominant) hand spread up her arm. After a couple of weeks she lost control over her arm, and this left her unable to write or to use her hand for any fine movements. Over a period of three months Ann felt weak and was chronically tired.

She learnt she had multiple sclerosis. She was a physiotherapist and well understood what the condition might mean. Yet this professional knowledge could not prepare her for the reality of confronting and living with the condition. Although her symptoms were relatively minor in medical terms, Ann felt that her life had been derailed. Confronted with the radical uncertainty of her condition and what the future would bring, her relationship with herself and her world was fundamentally altered.

The focus in this section will be on the research findings that relate to Ann's sense of bodily experience (embodiment) and her relations with others (sociality) during her first three months of coming to terms with the diagnosis.

EMBODIMENT: ALIENATED YET INESCAPABLE

With her fatigue, the loss of sensation in her arm and coordination problems, Ann experiences a disruption in her self-body-world, hitherto unified. Her ongoing engagement with the world – in phenomenological terms, her bodily intentionality – is thwarted as she can no longer do things she has previously taken for granted. Ann experiences her body as being alienated, out of control and inescapable.

In the first three months after the diagnosis, Ann comes to see her right arm as an 'it': 'It had a life of its own . . . it just used to fall off things . . . it would just suddenly come up like this and it was very strange.' That Ann can no longer feel the connection between herself and the world adds to a profound sense of bodily alienation.

A powerful reminder of this sense of alienation comes when she reaches out to touch – and be touched by – her children, only to discover that she cannot feel them. 'It is precisely my body which perceives the body of another person,' Merleau-Ponty (1962, p. 354) reminds us. And suddenly Ann has lost a significant connection with her children. 'Initially, it was difficult giving the children a proper cuddle which was just so terrible!' She panics at the thought of not being able to do the 'mummy thing' and feel the 'softness of their skin properly'. Without sensation, she loses her ability to caress and hold and to express her love. All her intimate relations are disrupted as her ability to embody her loving presence is thwarted.

At the same time, Ann has an acute awareness of inescapable embodiment. She cannot, however much she wants to, disassociate herself from her malfunctioning body. She has to cope with her life despite her body feeling fatigued. She cannot separate her arm from herself. As she rails 'Why me?' she is confronted by the truth that the multiple sclerosis is in her: it **is** her. She is forced to negotiate with her arm and gradually learn to incorporate it, in its altered state, back into herself.

With her arm desensitised and spatially dislocated, she has to learn how to carry out everyday living tasks (for herself and her children) in new and unfamiliar ways. Certain gestures are no longer within her bodily scope and her possibilities for action shrink. She learns a new way of *being-in-the-world* (Heidegger, 1962) where her eyes and arm work together to engage in daily living tasks. Ann describes her difficulty with doing up the buttons on her children's clothes: 'I have to watch, visually do it . . . it is much more difficult.' She notes, with an embarrassed laugh, that her own personal care also presents problems.

For example, she has to learn how to wipe herself with her other hand after going to the toilet.

Ann experiences her body ambivalently. Her arm is something both *a-part from* and *a-part of* herself. Here, we can usefully draw the distinction between the subjective body (as experienced pre-reflectively) and objective body (as observed and scientifically investigated).

For Ann, her pre-reflectively lived subjective body is disconnected. The comfortably familiar, taken-for-granted body that represents her continuing perspective on the world (what Sartre (1969) poetically calls the body 'passed-over-in-silence') now contains both an absence and a new, unfamiliar aspect. Her old arm is no longer there and she feels this loss acutely. For one thing, it has meant that she has had to give up her special hobby of doing fine needlework. But there is also a sense of a new presence. She has gained a new appendage: an 'it', an unseeable, unpredictable attacker, who does things without her volition. It feels out of her control, as if an alien infiltration has arbitrarily taken over and might suddenly turn round and 'kick [her] in the face again'. 'It' is the enemy, one called multiple sclerosis, which forced itself into her consciousness and took away her life as she knew it. Her task is to resist and subdue the enemy.

At the same time, Ann's arm is part of her objective body – one that she can observe, examine and feel disconnected from. Each morning she runs through the different parts of her body, checking they are still there and assessing her functioning. She evaluates her levels of fatigue and energy. She views her body with a medical gaze. With her professional understandings of multiple sclerosis she 'sees' the myelin sheaths of her peripheral nerves being eroded away. She assesses her own physical functioning as she has assessed that of others and as others have assessed her. The sick person understands and reflects on their experience through concepts derived from, and defined by, others – in Ann's case the medical profession. Sartre (1969) refers to this process as 'being-for-others'.

Yet even as she 'splits' off her body she also seeks to reconnect with her body. Her morning ritual 'check' offers a way of simultaneously embracing both her subjective and her objective body. As she runs through her body parts and assesses her functioning level for that day, she is affirming her body identity as a-part of herself, a-part from herself. 'The body, aware of itself in being aware of the world, stands in a relation "of embrace" with the world . . . Each morning I awake to "that blending with the world that recommences for me . . . as soon as

I open my eyes"' (Merleau-Ponty, 1968, paraphrased by Wider, 1997, p. 138).

SOCIALITY: TRYING TO 'PASS' – A SECRET SHAME?

For Ann, the loss of her capacity to touch and be touched disrupts her entire relational world. Yet even as her self–other relationships are under threat, Ann is engaged in a mission to try to minimise the impact. She tries to keep things as 'normal' as possible – she doesn't want the MS to contaminate her life. One way she does this is to split off her multiple sclerosis identity and keep it hidden, keep it secret. That people often conceal their illness from a society that does not understand is quite frequently encountered in the literature on disability (e.g. Miller, 1997).

After receiving the diagnosis, she does not want to tell anyone – even her husband. Multiple sclerosis is something she has to cope with alone (and she is used to coping alone, as her husband is away much of the time). While not denying her diagnosis to herself, she consciously seeks to protect others – particularly her children and husband. Over the course of a few weeks Ann's husband slowly becomes aware of the situation, though they still do not discuss the condition openly. 'I just sort of led him gently,' she says. 'I gradually dripped it in and removed any other options . . . I just felt it was better for him . . . he copes with things better that way.' While she slowly begins to disclose the diagnosis to a couple of friends and her sisters, her way of coping generally is to protect others from the horror of her experience.

So this multiple sclerosis side is a part of herself that is somehow unrecognised in public: it is untalked to. This self only emerges when she is alone in bed at night. Here she confronts her existential aloneness. She cries and rages, but these tears are shared only with her self. Her husband and children are shielded from her vulnerability and mortality. Ann copes by throwing herself into her mother role and trying to preserve what she can of it. At the same time she gives up her work and hobbies. It seems as though she has chosen one role to do well. And her mother role is centrally important to her. In a way, her children are an extension of her own identity.

In her mother role, Ann is engaged in an urgent mission to keep things 'normal'. She seeks to continue caring for her children and to preserve a sense of continuity as a 'mummy-who-is-there'. In the face of her own insecurity, she seeks to do all she can to ensure her children's security. This pattern whereby sufferers strive to maintain 'normal' functioning by minimising or disguising their symptoms has been described by Charmaz (2000), along with others.

The mission to keep things normal also seeps into Ann's other relationships. Here, she tries to 'pass' as the old Ann. Somehow, she gains a sense of stability from people reacting to her as they always have. She doesn't want to build relationships on the basis of their pity, or with them focusing on just this one aspect of her, judging and stereotyping her. In a sense, Ann is working hard to minimise changes, or threats, to her relations with others. She hides her multiple sclerosis so that it doesn't 'contaminate' things. She seems to fear the feelings of shame that may engulf her as she stands in the 'gaze' of the Other. Ann doesn't want to be revealed to herself as a multiple sclerosis sufferer through the looks of others. Through that 'look' she is objectified and so experiences shame (Sartre, 1969). As Toombs explains:

> One sees one's disordered body style through the eyes of the Other . . . This is not a culture that celebrates physical difference or dependence . . . Every time I have had to adopt a new way of getting around the world . . . I have experienced feelings of shame. (Toombs, 2001, p. 257)

REFLECTIONS

In this section I aim to evaluate my study **reflexively** (Finlay and Gough, 2003). First, I explore the role Ann played in the co-construction of my findings while arguing against the use of participants to 'validate' research. I then offer some reflections on the strengths and limitations of my research and methodology.

PARTICIPANT COLLABORATION, NOT VALIDATION

Ann and I collaborated in this research in a number of ways. First of all, she agreed to share her experience with me as she was keen that I 'spread the word' to therapists about what it was 'really like to have MS'. Together, we embarked on a project whose findings, we both understood, would eventually be made public. Ann was content for me to share the findings with therapists. That the interviews were conducted in a natural conversation style helped foster that sense of collaboration. As I moved on to analyse the interviews I consulted Ann several times, discussing with her my perceptions and analysis. In these ways Ann can be said to have played a part in co-constituting the findings.

As Ann was a physiotherapist she had a reasonable understanding of the aims, process and intended outcomes of my case-study research. This was important, as it meant that her consent to take part in the research was properly informed. It also meant that Ann could take on a more collaborative role in the research to the extent that she wanted to. In a spirit of openness, I left this decision to her. While she wanted an opportunity for discussion, she seemed content to hand authorial control to me, understanding that this would be my research. As a health professional, Ann was interested to discuss both the findings of my broader study and my analysis of her particular interview. I was pleased to share my findings with her. In return, she offered me her reactions.

Ann was particularly active on hearing my preliminary analysis of the interviews with her. She affirmed certain themes, suggesting I had captured her experience 'nicely'. At other points she suggested that my analysis (particularly my metaphorical flourishes) needed to be 'toned down' as she didn't feel they represented her ordinary, everyday experience. One notable example here was my initial use of an analogy: that of Ann's situation being akin to 'living with an alien monster'. I rather liked this metaphor, regarding it as both punchy and poetic, and was reluctant to let it go. However, it was not something Ann could relate to. I therefore deleted all references to the monster while retaining (I ruefully acknowledge) some sense of the notion of alien infiltration.

In retrospect, I can see that it was useful to get Ann's feedback. For one thing, it helped me to better appreciate how Ann had, in fact, managed to reconnect with her 'disconnected' arm. I remain uncomfortably aware that our collaboration was partial and not entirely mutual. While Ann gave me some feedback, I retained control of my analysis and writing. In the end it is I who was choosing where, when, what and how to publish the findings. And, in the end, these are my findings, my interpretations. I could have involved Ann much more collaboratively, but chose not to.

That Ann has been somewhat involved in the co-production of my findings perhaps strengthens the trustworthiness and ethical base of this research. However, I stop short of claiming that Ann has 'validated' this study in any way. I do not seek a 'truth' that can be validated in this way. Instead, I tend towards a more relativist position, one recognising that my findings have emerged in a specific context, that my telling of Ann's story is specific to the time, place and individuals concerned. Another researcher working with Ann would have unfolded a different story. So most likely would I, had I undertaken the research at a different point in time or in different circumstances.

Many qualitative researchers embrace the idea of 'participant validation' as a way to 'prove' the validity of their research. When the participant agrees with the researcher's assessment, it is seen as strengthening the researcher's argument. Such confidence, however, may be misplaced. It needs to be remembered that participants have their own motives, needs and interests, to say nothing of varying degrees of insight. Further, what may have been 'true' for them at the time of the interview may no longer be the case. Their ability to put themselves back into the specific research context may be limited. In his critical exploration of participant validation, Ashworth (1993) supports it on moral-political grounds, but warns against taking participants' evaluations too seriously: it may be in their interest to protect their 'socially presented selves'. As he notes, 'Participant validation is flawed nevertheless, since the "atmosphere of safety" that would allow the individual to lower his or her defences, cease "presentation", and act in open candour (if this is possible), is hardly likely to be achieved in the research encounter' (Ashworth, 1993, p. 15).

EVALUATION OF THE RESEARCH

In this chapter I have focused selectively on two key existential themes in order to demonstrate the nature of phenomenological description and writing. Space has not permitted the inclusion of many quotes and illustrative examples that would have helped provide a fuller, more transparent account of my reasoning and interpretation. The strength and special contribution of the phenomenological method lies in the way it can capture the richness, complexity, ambiguity and ambivalence of lived experience. The quality of any phenomenological study can be judged through its ability to share its discoveries, to draw the reader ever deeper into the worlds of others. I believe that my study of Ann's experience has gone some way to achieving this.

Polkinghorne (1983) offers four qualities to help the reader judge the power and trustworthiness of phenomenological accounts: vividness, accuracy, richness and elegance. Is the research vivid in the sense that it generates a sense of reality and draws the reader in? Are readers able to recognise the phenomenon from their own experience or from imagining the situation vicariously? In terms of richness, can readers enter the account emotionally? Finally, has the phenomenon been described in a graceful, clear, poignant way?

I would argue that I have, indeed, glimpsed something of Ann's perceptions and her world and that my findings do resonate with her 'real' (or, at least, her perceived) experience. However, my findings remain partial, tentative and emergent. If we accept that the phenomenological method involves interpretation of meanings, it follows that any one analysis can only be presented as a 'tentative statement opening upon a limitless field of possible interpretations' (Churchill, 2000, p. 164). In making these claims, I am placing myself somewhere between a critical realist and a relativist epistemological position.

In common with any qualitative approach, phenomenological findings cannot easily be generalised to wider populations. I claim only to have described something of Ann's particular experience, not the experience of multiple sclerosis generally. The phenomenon I have sought to describe is to be understood not as something with an objective reference point, but rather as something that occurs for one individual (in this case, Ann) in the context of her specific meanings and situation. At the same time, I would expect the findings to resonate with others who have multiple sclerosis. Therein lies the particular potency of phenomenological research.

In conclusion, the findings from my research show something of how the diagnosis of multiple sclerosis creates a sense of global uncertainty that permeates Ann's being. That she can no longer be certain what her physical condition will be tomorrow or next year threatens her dreams of the future and disrupts her relations with herself and others in the now. Her response is to throw herself into being a good mother. She copes to some extent by compartmentalising and seeking the oasis of ('hyper')-normality. As her life is derailed, it is also being reclaimed and actively worked. As she begins to adjust to her diagnosis she is reconnecting with her alienated body. She is managing to subdue and learn to live with her body, which is not quite in her control. What is a-part *from* herself is becoming a-part *of* herself.

With this sort of existential-phenomenological analysis, the focus is on describing – trying to 'bring to life' – a participant's immediate lived experience. The strength of this method is its ability to capture the richness of people's existence through describing ordinary, mundane living. And yet, when we focus so deeply on aspects of individuals' ordinary lives, what is revealed is, inevitably, something special; something *more*. What is revealed is, in fact, quite extraordinary.

REFERENCES

Ashworth, P.D. (1993) 'Participant agreement in the justification of qualitative findings', *Journal of Phenomenological Psychology*, 24: 3–16.

Ashworth, P. (2003) 'An approach to phenomenological psychology: The contingencies of the lifeworld', *Journal of Phenomenological Psychology*, 34(6): 145–56.

Bury, M. (1982) 'Chronic illness as biographical disruption', *Sociology of Health and Illness*, 4(2): 167–82.

Charmaz, K. (2000) 'Experiencing chronic illness', in Albrecht, G.L., Fitzpatrick, R. and Scrimshaw, S.C. (eds), *The Handbook of Social Studies in Health and Medicine*, London: Sage Publications.

Churchill, S.D. (2000) 'Phenomenological psychology', in Kazdin, A.D. (ed.), *Encyclopedia of Psychology*, Oxford: Oxford University Press.

Finlay, L. (1999) 'Applying phenomenology in research: Problems, principles and practice', *British Journal of Occupational Therapy*, 62(7): 299–306.

Finlay, L. (2005) 'Reflexive embodied empathy: A phenomenology of participant–researcher intersubjectivity', *The Humanistic Psychologist*, 33(4): 271–92.

Finlay, L. and Gough, B. (eds) (2003) *Reflexivity: A Practical Guide for Researchers in Health and Social Sciences*, Oxford: Blackwell Publishing.

Frank, A.W. (1995) *The Wounded Story Teller: Body, Illness and Ethics*, Chicago: University of Chicago Press.

Giorgi, A. (ed.) (1985) *Phenomenology and Psychological Research*, Pittsburgh, PA: Duquesne University Press.

Heidegger, M. (1962) *Being and Time* (trans. J. Macquarrie and E. Robinson), New York: Harper and Row (original work published 1927).

Husserl, E. (1970) *The Crisis of European Sciences and Transcendental Phenomenology*, Evanston, IL: Northwestern University Press.

Koopman, W. and Schweitzer, A. (1999) 'The journey to multiple sclerosis: A qualitative study', *Journal of Neuroscience Nursing*, 31(1): 17–26.

Merleau-Ponty, M. (1962) *Phenomenology of Perception* (trans. C. Smith), London: Routledge & Kegan Paul (original work published 1945).

Merleau-Ponty, M. (1968) *The Visible and the Invisible* (trans. A. Lingis). Evanston, IL: Northwestern University Press (original work published 1964).

Miller, C.M. (1997) 'Relapsing multiple sclerosis: A phenomenological study', *Journal of Neuroscience Nursing*, 29(5): 294–304.

Polkinghorne, D. (1983) *Methodology for the Human Sciences*, Albany: Suny Press.

Rogers, C.R. (1975) 'Empathic: An unappreciated way of being', *Counselling Psychologist*, 5(20): 2–10.

Sartre, J.-P. (1969) *Being and Nothingness* (trans. H. Barnes), London: Routledge (original work published 1943).

Toombs, S.K. (1995) 'Sufficient unto the day: A life with multiple sclerosis', in Toombs, S.K., Barnard, D. and Carson, R. (eds), *Chronic Illness: From Experience to Policy*, Bloomington/Indianapolis: Indiana University Press.

Toombs, S.K. (2001) 'Reflections on bodily change: The lived experience of disability', in Toombs, S.K. (ed.), *Phenomenology and Medicine*, Dordrecht, Holland: Kluwer Academic Publishers.

Valle, R.S. and Halling, S. (eds) (1989) *Existential Phenomenological Perspectives in Psychology: Exploring the Breadth of Human Experience*, New York: Plenum.

van Manen, M. (1990) *Researching Lived Experience: Human Science for an Action Sensitive Pedagogy*, New York: State University of New York Press.

Wertz, F.J. (1983) 'From everyday to psychological description: Analyzing the moments of a qualitative data analysis', *Journal of Phenomenological Psychology*, 14(2): 197–241.

Wider, K.V. (1997) *The Bodily Nature of Consciousness*, London: Cornell University Press.

ACKNOWLEDGEMENTS

Special thanks go to Fred Wertz, Editor, for allowing me to reproduce material from Finlay, L. (2003) 'The intertwining of body, self and world: A phenomenological study of living with recently diagnosed multiple sclerosis', *Journal of Phenomenological Psychology*, 34(2): 157–78.

14

Discourse Analysis in Action: The Construction of Risk in a Community Day Hospital

CLAIRE BALLINGER AND JULIANNE CHEEK

In this chapter, we explore how discourse analysis (DA) influenced by postmodern/poststructural thought can be used to explore and challenge aspects of health care provision. We begin by outlining what we understand discourse analysis (as influenced by such theoretical frames) to be. Drawing on the work of Parker (1992), we then highlight some strategies that can guide research using this approach. We demonstrate these strategies in action by drawing on a study of how risk is constructed and understood within the context of a community day hospital for older people. In so doing, our aim is not to provide a definitive answer as to what discourse analysis is, but rather to open up the concept of discourse analysis for scrutiny and offer one way in which research employing it might be shaped.

METHODOLOGY: TOWARDS UNDERSTANDING DISCOURSE ANALYSIS

While discourse analysis remains relatively under-represented in the allied health research literature, it has been gaining prominence within the general field of qualitative research, conducted across a variety of

Qualitative Research for Allied Health Professionals: Challenging Choices. Edited by Linda Finlay and Claire Ballinger.   Copyright 2006 by John Wiley & Sons Ltd.   ISBN 0-470-01963-8.

academic disciplines. However, as it has increased in popularity, confusion about its purpose, ontology and methods has, if anything, intensified. Part of the confusion stems from the fact that discourse analysis is not a unified approach, so it is important to both understand and articulate which approach to discourse analysis is in play in any piece of research.

The theoretical perspectives that we are drawing on in this chapter stem from postmodern and poststructural understandings of reality. Rather than seeking universal and essential truths, postmodern thought recognises 'the existence of multiple perspectives, assuming instead plurality of understandings for any aspect of social reality' (Cheek, 2000, p. 19). The work of the French philosopher Michel Foucault has been consistently associated with this perspective, though he himself resisted such categorisation, preferring to describe his work as a 'history of the present' (Foucault, 1977, p. 31). Foucault problematised knowledge by challenging the notion that 'knowledge is objective and value-free, inevitably progressive, and universal' (Cheek, 2000, p. 22). Rather, Foucault posited the intimate association between power and knowledge (e.g. 1975, 1977) and explored this 'power/knowledge' link using his concept of discourse. Discourse, he argued, was a way of thinking about reality that both **enables** and **excludes**. It enables what can be said or thought at any point in time while at the same time operating to exclude or marginalise other ways of viewing reality. As Kress neatly summarises, Foucault's understanding of discourse 'provides a set of possible statements about a given area, and organises and gives structure to the manner in which a particular topic, object, process is to be talked about' (Kress, 1985, p. 7).

Within health, much has been written about how medical knowledge and practices have shaped the ways in which the body is known, how certain practices come to be defined as appropriate and authoritative and how health and illness more generally are understood. In contemporary health care, medical/scientific discourse has achieved a 'truth' status in which many underpinning premises and assumptions about health care are neither recognised nor questioned. A current example is that of vaccination. Great effort has been expended by governments in the UK, Australasia and the USA to increase the numbers of people, especially children, seeking vaccination against major diseases such as measles. In order to add to the legitimacy of these campaigns, the accounts of medical experts have been used to add support to the pro-immunisation message. In contrast, those wary of, or opposed to, certain forms of inoculation have been represented in ways that emphasise their 'otherness' and challenge the credibility of this 'alternate' perspective (Dew, 1999).

An important point here is that, in contrast to a Marxist perspective, Foucault did not view power as necessarily a repressive force that is held by one person or group. He saw it as the inevitable consequence of sociohistoric processes that enable different discourses to assume dominance at different times – this is why Foucault calls himself a historian of the present. Power, argued Foucault, is intimately linked to the ways in which we know, understand and represent everyday experiences. There is a dynamic relationship between power and knowledge in that the knowledge that underpins a discourse is used by proponents of that discourse to claim presence and exclude other. It is the operation of such webs of power that enable certain knowledge to be produced and 'known'. Power, therefore, in such analysis is not just repressive but also productive. Which discourses are prominent at any particular point in time in history is an effect of the outworking of power/knowledge. Discursive frameworks order reality in a particular way, rendering it visible and understandable. At the same time, they constrain the production of understanding and knowledge that might offer alternate views of that reality.

The task of the discourse analyst is to make explicit the ways in which discourses operate within particular contexts. They ask such questions as: How have these particular discourses arisen? What is assumed or implicit in their use? What versions of reality do they construct and sustain? Do contesting discourses exist? How are dominant discourses maintained? How does the version of reality that they sustain mesh with discourses at work within other contexts?

We now turn to clarify some key principles and features of discourse analysis informed by postmodern/poststructural perspectives.

SYSTEMATIC AND EXPLICIT ANALYSIS

A fundamental principle of discourse analysis is that texts are analysed in a systematic and explicit fashion. One of the problems in some reports of studies purporting to use discourse analysis, is that neither the underpinning approach, nor the way in which it has been used have been clarified. The rather vague epistemological position of the researcher and nonspecific mode of analysis then tend to be equated with difficulties with this methodology itself, rather than viewed as an example of poor scholarship.

A challenge to the novice researcher wishing to carry out a discourse analysis is that descriptions of 'how to do it' are difficult to find. Parker (1992) argues against providing recipes or steps for researchers to follow, highlighting that our interests and values are intimately connected with our research approach. He argues that to view research methods as 'value-free tools' that can be adopted and used by anyone is to bring an atheoretical stance to bear on the research venture. We concur with this view, arguing that researchers need to ground themselves thoroughly in the theoretical underpinnings of the approach to discourse analysis that they are using. When appraising a discourse analytic study, we suggest looking for evidence of such grounding from the theorists and texts that are cited to situate the approach taken. Within this chapter, for example, we acknowledge the work of Foucault (1975, 1977) in respect of broad postmodern/poststructural orientation to discourse analysis, and draw more specifically from the writings and work of Parker (1992, 1994). We, the chapter authors, acknowledge these theorists as informing our understandings of discourse analysis. We also acknowledge the influence of Lupton (1997) and Armstrong (1997) on our characterisation of a scientific/biomedical discourse.

ANALYSIS OF TEXTS

The basic unit of analysis within discourse analysis is the text. Data collection in discourse analysis involves the generation and/or collection of texts to which a discursive lens can be applied. Parker describes this as 'treating our objects of study as texts which are described, put into words' (1992, p. 3). Textual data of interest to discourse analysts in allied health might include patient information leaflets, newspaper reports or medical notes. They might also be derived from dialogue: for example conversations and research interviews, in which talk is audio or video recorded and transcribed, in common with many other qualitative approaches. Yet other texts might be derived from observations that are then recorded as fieldnotes.

In a study by the second author (JC) on media representations of toxic shock syndrome (TSS), media articles referring to the syndrome were collected as texts for analysis (Cheek, 1997). These texts were interrogated using discourse analytic principles to expose the discursive frameworks that have an impact on how this syndrome is represented within the media. This article provides an example of a form of discourse analysis in action.

TEXT AS PRODUCTIVE

A third principle of discourse analysis (at least within the particular analytic approach we are exploring here) is that texts are not viewed as neutral ways of conveying information. Instead, they are understood as playing a crucial role in the construction of particular versions of reality. To a discourse analyst drawing on Foucauldian understandings of discourse, the assumptions that the text makes 'in presuming that it will be understood' (Agger, 1991, p. 112) are of as much interest as the topic or content. Texts are therefore productive, challenging notions of 'natural' or 'authentic' accounts of reality. For example, in the toxic shock syndrome study, discourse analysis highlighted that the medical/scientific discourse evident within the media articles reified this syndrome as a specific disease with recognised symptoms. Through the production of this particular version of reality, other experiences, which did not fit with this norm, could be rejected or marginalised (Cheek, 1997).

SITUATING TEXTS IN THEIR SOCIAL, CULTURAL, POLITICAL AND HISTORICAL CONTEXTS

Another principle of discourse analysis is its focus on how particular texts are indicative of wider cultural understandings and ways of sense making. Consider the following headline, from the toxic shock syndrome (TSS) study referred to previously:

'Scary' new disease kills women

This headline and the associated article appeared in 1980 on the front page of *The Advertiser*, a daily newspaper in the state of South Australia. This was the first time that TSS had been reported in this paper.

Cheek (2000, p. 104) asks a number of questions of this headline, which challenge its status as neutral reporting, while encouraging consideration of its wider cultural contexts:

- Why was the word 'scary' used and not another word?
- What connotations does the word 'scary' have?
- TSS is referred to as a 'new disease'. Where does this locate TSS and how will such a location affect the way TSS is viewed by women, health professionals and others?

The tone of the headline is one of shock – 'scary' in inverted commas contrasts with the more formal language that follows. The shock value is reinforced when one realises that the word 'scary' is a direct quote from the woman doctor acting as the spokesperson for the US-based Federal Center for Disease Control; a doctor, one supposes, is someone who would not normally make use of rather emotive language. The word 'scary' carries connotations of childhood 'scary' stories or situations. It thereby positions TSS as something warranting a fearful response, which renders one small and powerless, like a child confronting the unknown. Through the use of the word 'disease', TSS is placed firmly within a medical context, within the realms of doctors, patients, signs and symptoms – in short, a scientific and rational location. TSS thus becomes something that ordinary women cannot hope to manage themselves; they need to seek advice and help from experts who operate within this scientific/medical context.

This example, and the study of which it is part, draws attention to the performative qualities of texts. They demonstrate how the use of particular words, and types of words, reveals implicit and unstated understandings within the text(s) that draw on different discursive frames.

DOING THE RESEARCH: DISCOURSE ANALYTIC STRATEGIES IN ACTION

INTERROGATING THE DATA

In this section we use a specific piece of research to demonstrate discourse analysis in action. The research was carried out by the first author (CB) within the context of a community day hospital for older people. The aim of the study was to explore how understandings of risk were constructed and used within this environment. The study was carried out following a smaller-scale exploration of the perspectives of older people and therapists on risk specifically related to falls and falling. See Ballinger (1999) and Ballinger and Payne (2002) for a fuller account of the analysis.

Three methods of generating texts were used: participant observation within the community day hospital, interviews with older service users, and collection of documents including the operational policy of the day hospital and copies of information leaflets and booklets produced for service users.

The fieldnotes, interview transcripts and documents as texts were then interrogated, drawing on Parker (1992), by asking the following questions of the texts:

- What kind of visual images are conjured up by the texts?
- What kinds of people are present in the world alluded to or described within the texts? How about the people least likely to be associated with this world?
- What are the important things, ideas and/or tasks in the sort of world created by the texts? What type of world is conjured up by these texts?

Examples of asking each of these questions of specific texts in this study are now provided to illustrate discourse analysis in action.

What Kind of Visual Images Are Conjured up by the Texts?

One text collected in the study was an information booklet provided to new service users. This detailed the roles of the various health professionals in the community day hospital. It described the role of the nurse in this way:

> A **nurse** will be involved with specific nursing care such as well-person checks, monitoring of blood pressure, management of continence, and monitoring of medication. (bold text in original)

This directive evokes a rather mechanistic image of a nurse tending to a patient in a rather similar fashion to a mechanic attending to a car during a yearly service, checking oil or testing tyre pressure. Checking, monitoring and managing are to the fore, with the person being examined not visible apart from as the object on which these things will be carried out. Excerpts from observational fieldnotes and interviews conducted by CB reinforced this. Here is part of a conversation with a new attendee whom CB had not met before:

> She told me that it was her first day, and a doctor had examined her very thoroughly: 'There was not a part of my body that wasn't asked about' (dhvis22 lines 105–9)

In this woman's account of her first day at the day hospital, there appeared to be little interest in her as a person: how she was feeling or how she perceived her problems. Rather, as with the description of the role of the nurse, the focus was on checking and monitoring how her body as object was functioning, reinforcing a mechanistic, objective way of viewing this woman.

Another excerpt, taken from fieldnotes, records a discussion between two physiotherapy staff, one of whom held a list of names:

She had put initials by the names of all the people to be treated by the physios and told (the Senior Physiotherapist) 'I've done Mrs Smith' (dhvis15 lines 443–7)

'Done' is an interesting word for her to use. Contrast this way of communicating with these alternatives: 'I have worked with Mrs Smith', 'Mrs Smith has been seen', or 'Mrs Smith has received her treatment'. The use of 'done' reinforces the notion of people waiting to be serviced or processed.

What Kinds of People Are Present in the World Alluded to or Described within the Texts? How about the People Least Likely to be Associated with this World?

The texts generated in this study construct a world in which people are positioned and defined by the way health care practice is understood and carried out in the day hospital. Health care staff possess **expert knowledge** about the body, disease and the means of alleviating or curing the resulting problems. Assessment and monitoring comprise an important part of such expert knowledge, both in terms of having the authority to carry out the assessment, and also in terms of the knowledge that the assessment provides. Staff also decide on best treatment, and ultimately how long an individual needs to attend the day hospital. The service users, or patients, by contrast, are relatively inactive. Their role is to attend, act in accordance with recommendations and, where appropriate, practise new skills at home.

During an interview, a service user described a physiotherapy session that had occurred some weeks previously:

because (the physiotherapists) said they'd let me practise the lot so that I could walk if the doctor wanted me to . . . he didn't . . . he just felt my knee or worked my knee and inspected the scar and he said everything was fine . . . and I've had x-rays and he said they were good so I didn't have to walk for the doctor after all (s2p3 lines 292–311)

In this excerpt, the physiotherapists appear to be preparing the service user for assessment by the doctor. The service user positions herself as passive and compliant – 'they'd let me', 'if the doctor wanted me to'. As she describes the incident, there is no room or role for her own contribution about her progress. It is the doctor who says that 'everything was fine' – with 'everything' here presumably referring to the physical healing process as determined by medical discourse.

Similarly, the service user describes a situation where she seems to have little if any say in what occurs in the interaction with the doctor – she was prepared to walk if required, but the doctor simply performed some physical tests, declared that progress was satisfactory and did not call on her to demonstrate her mobility. Note, too, the importance attached to medical technology here: the X-rays are held to show that healing had taken place – 'they were good' – and this means that no further dialogue, discussion or demonstration was deemed necessary.

Within the world described by this service user, it would be difficult to imagine her refusing to let the doctor touch her knee. It is unlikely that she would communicate her views about her own lack of progress or contradict the doctor's judgement. Those able to use technology and possessing the knowledge to understand the intimate workings of the body are positioned as expert. Patients like this woman cannot contribute to such understandings. Consequently, they are not afforded a voice in interactions drawing on these frames. Although present as object (in this case as 'the knee') they are absent as person. A very different interaction might have occurred if the woman was asked how she felt about her knee surgery and what it might mean for her in her everyday life. She, as person, would not be absent from this conversation or frame.

An important point to note in discourse analysis of this type is that texts are not seen primarily as records of events or as illustrations of the speaker's beliefs or attitudes. The primary interest lies in the way such texts construct a particular worldview by what they include, what is absent from them and how the players are positioned.

What Are the Important Things, Ideas and/or Tasks in the Sort of World Created by the Texts? What Type of World Is Conjured up by these Texts?

We have already noted that the texts cited seem to foreground technical skills requiring expert knowledge and sometimes specialist equipment (e.g. X-rays, blood-pressure monitors). Within this world of the day hospital, people are recognised through their capacity to perform specialised and specific tasks. It is a world in which individuals are positioned in relation to particular forms of knowledge and the authority that such knowledge is used to claim. Consider the following fieldnote about how the housekeeper characterises her role within the day hospital:

(The housekeeper) asked if I had been at (the General Hospital), and explained that her role as housekeeper was different to the cleaners at (the General Hospital). She has responsibility for checking people in, doing things with their food; she explained that it was difficult to get the thickener right and she had to note if they were diabetic. (dhvis2 lines 70–79)

Of the various jobs that the housekeeper completes on a daily basis, she chooses to outline her tasks related to the preparation of meals. She emphasises that such preparation ensures that no untoward medical events such as aspiration occur, as well as the provision of appropriate meals for service users with diabetes. She distinguishes herself from those with cleaning roles at other hospitals through the identification of the specialist tasks that she has responsibility for completing. She is laying claim to a particular form of expertise.

The things, objects or concepts that are not present within the worlds constructed by the texts are also of interest. They might be absent because they are not understood, have no purpose or are viewed as being of lesser importance or significance. Thus it is interesting that the housekeeper does not identify providing meals that the service users enjoy and find pleasurable as being an important part of her role. Rather, she draws on a specific discourse, the dominant discursive frame in the world in which she operates, to describe what she does and what she understands her world to be about. Thus when using discourse analysis it can be useful to ask: Who/what is not present? Which objects or concepts is it difficult to imagine or make a case for in the world of the text?

Within the world of the day hospital constructed so far, one of the features that has been absent has been the voice of the service user, actively contributing to the espoused purpose of the day hospital and the framing of their needs within this context. Foucault's link between power/knowledge is important here: only those with specialist knowledge or expertise can lay claim to authority and status within the construction that is the day hospital. As illustrated in the example of the woman who was having her knee examined, users of the service who generally lack detailed knowledge of anatomy and pathology are positioned as having little to contribute to their own recovery. Their own views about their progress, motivation to recover and support at home are in general not seen as relevant in a setting premised on scientific/medical understandings.

FINDINGS: RISK AS CONSTRUCTED WITHIN SCIENTIFIC/BIOMEDICAL DISCOURSE

The structure outlined by the editors of this book asked for a section of each of the Part II chapters to address the findings of the research being discussed. To label any one point in a discourse analytic process as 'findings' is misleading: the entire process produces insights or 'findings'. For example, the discussion in the previous section analyses ways in which the study setting is discursively constructed. This paves the way for, and is central to, exploring how risk is spoken and thought about in this setting. After much thought and debate, in order to be consistent with other chapters in this book, we have called this section 'findings'. We do so at this point of the discussion because we have reached the stage within our discourse analysis when we start to identify discourses present within the texts we are interrogating. Having done so, we are able to move on to attempt to understand how these discursive frames affect understandings of risk, given that the aim of the study we are using to demonstrate discourse in action was to explore the way risk is understood in a day community hospital. Working within these parameters we now interrogate the texts generated in this study asking: What are the discourses that are present within these texts, and what shall we name them? We return to our feelings of unease about the use of the term 'findings' in the reflections section of this chapter.

Given the space constraints of this chapter, and the fact that the study as a whole has been reported elsewhere (Ballinger and Payne, 2002), we will focus on one of the discourses to emerge from our analysis. This we term scientific/biomedical discourse. Other discourses operate to frame risk, for example legal and managerial discourses. In common with the 'medical/scientific' discourse described by Cheek (2000), 'scientific/biomedical discourse', as we have highlighted in earlier sections of this chapter, focuses on the objectified body. Commentators such as Lupton (1994) and Armstrong (1995, 1997), drawing on the writings of Foucault (1975, 1977), have written about the objectified body as it is wrought through medical texts and practices, classified, categorised and subject to scrutiny, both external and internal, using technologies such as the X-rays and blood tests used in our study setting. Other features of this discourse include the privileging of expert knowledge about the body and its systems over lay accounts about how disease or illness are manifest in the lives of those in whom they are present (Lupton, 1994).

We have already surfaced examples of this in earlier analyses of the study setting.

By naming this frame scientific/biomedical discourse we are emphasising the role of science in informing a view of health care that has in its main frame a view of medicine that emphasises the role of physical science and attendant technical skills, as opposed to, for example, a view of medicine where a more holistic view is present, or a view of health care where medicine is not in the main frame at all.

However, the identification of a discourse, or discourses, does not mark the end of the discourse analysis. It provides us with the means to ask yet more pertinent and interesting questions, such as:

- How are particular sorts of individuals, organisations and systems legitimised and strengthened through the operation of certain discourses?
- How do discourses work together to sustain particular realities and truths?

As has been demonstrated, scientific/biomedical discourse foregrounds expert knowledge about the body, and highlights the role of health care professionals in diagnosing sickness and disease and deciding on appropriate medical care. Older service users – 'patients' – are positioned within the discourse as bearers of disease or lesions and the objects of medical assessment and intervention. The day hospital is constructed as an organisational setting designed to manage malfunctions present in older bodies by giving patients access to personnel with appropriate knowledge and relevant medical technology. Thus a system is created for managing these medical 'problems', and the positions of those who lay claim to expertise based on relevant power/knowledge are reinforced and strengthened.

With respect to constructions of risk, such scientific/biomedical discourse perpetuates the expert role of the doctor/health professional by entrusting them with the identification of 'risky agents' using the apparatus of science in the form of tests and procedures. It also enables these experts to claim authority in terms of the management of risk for this group of patients within the setting of the day hospital. The activity of walking serves well as an example. Several interview participants expressed an understanding, similar to that of the service user below, that patients were required to indicate to staff if they intended walking somewhere:

> they always wanted to make sure that you moved safely. That if you got up and tried to walk walk down to the toilets by yourself you'd be

virtually ticked off, you know you're not supposed to walk without somebody with you I was told. (ints2p2)

Framed within scientific/biomedical discourse, the act of walking is able
to be constructed as a risk. Once this has occurred it is possible to
monitor it, claim expertise about it and normalise it. Thus it is possible
to talk about safe and unsafe walking, including who can or cannot
walk, when, where and how. Hence, under the supervision of an expert
– a member of staff – and within the context of physiotherapy, 'risky'
walking becomes a 'safe' activity and a medium of treatment. However,
there are other situations where walking is able to be constructed as a
risky business and therefore proscriptions and constraints can be put
in place to minimise this constructed risk.

Nevertheless, it is not just risk as it relates to walking that is able to
be scrutinised and regulated. A variety of routines and procedures have
evolved to manage perceived dangers and risks in the day hospital
setting. On arrival, all patients were required to surrender to the
nursing staff any medication they needed to take during the day. The
staff kept this in a locked cupboard for administration by staff at intervals throughout the day. All patients were expected to adhere to this
rule whether or not they were responsible for taking their own medication at home, as indeed many were. Prepared meals were characterised as safe or unsafe for patients with diabetes. The names of those
with diabetes were listed in the kitchen in order to check which type
of meal people should be served. Separate desserts were prepared for
people with diabetes, and these individuals were served before everyone else. Many of those attending the day hospital prepared their own
meals at home, and those with diabetes would be used to making decisions about which foods they were able to eat. However, the effects of
scientific/biomedical discourse minimise patient agency, entrusting
responsibility instead to those held to possess the requisite medical
knowledge. Such discursive frames thereby reinforce the position of
the 'expert' staff while further disempowering patients, albeit often
consensually.

With the privileging of scientific/biomedical discourse in the day hospital setting, other characteristics of service users – including their own
preferences, capabilities and desires – fade into the background. The
reality of the day hospital becomes its capacity to monitor, assess and
rectify the body's workings. Objects deemed to be 'at risk' within this
discursive frame are of a physical or corporeal nature: bones at risk of
breaking, body systems at risk of damage through ingested toxins. Risks

arising from older people's concerns about social identities and roles, and risks resulting from stigmatising and infantilising practices, are not visible through the lens of scientific/biomedical discourse.

REFLECTIONS

Parker (1992) reminds us that the identification and naming of discourses involve 'moral/political' choices on the part of the analyst, encouraging the researcher to think reflexively about how they position themselves within these worlds. In the same way, writing a chapter about discourse analysis and the findings of a study and using it to explore understandings about risk in a community day hospital in the UK involves choices on the part of the authors with respect to what to put in the chapter in terms of content, but also how to structure the discussion. We have been employing a form of reflexivity throughout the writing and revising of this chapter that has forced both of us to think about what it is that we want to achieve and how best to do that. Such reflexivity also involved us thinking about how best to structure this reflections section. We have decided that a useful way might be to write about the things that often remain hidden or unspoken in reports of research – the decisions made and the dilemmas faced along the way. We write this in the form of a dialogue between us where we reflect on each other's reflections! My (CB) response to these dilemmas is self-consciously to note some of my challenges as I reflect back, while asking Julianne to provide an additional commentary that will trouble and act as a counterpoint to my unitary voice here.

CLAIRE   As I start to write this section, I feel myself once again shifting uncomfortably with the structure suggested for this chapter (albeit one that I was involved in identifying), and chafing against its perceived constraints. In this section, one is supposed to elegantly summarise one's responses to the chosen approach, highlight some useful reflections that might serve to help other researchers, and neatly end the chapter.

JULIANNE   Like Claire I have thought deeply about the best way to structure this chapter. For me it has been useful to remind myself that this chapter is as much a text as the data that we have used from the research study reported in it. As such, the chapter itself has understandings and assumptions embedded within it as to what a chapter is and how a chapter for a research methods book 'should' be written. It is assumptions about what a 'normal' research report might look like with prescribed linear sections that we have struggled against, in that we are discussing an approach to research in which all aspects of the research process are open to scrutiny and form part of the analysis. Further, it is impossible to offer a neat and single way of understanding discourse analysis. Given this, what we have been trying to do in this chapter is to open up readers' understandings to the plurality of approaches that are described as discourse analysis and emphasise the import-ance of situating one's approach within this diversity. It has not been to offer any sense of closure in a traditional sense by pro-viding a prescriptive way or series of steps to follow when doing discourse analysis.

CLAIRE   Initially I recall struggling with the discourse analysis liter-ature, as I tried to comprehend radically new ideas that challenged my previous ways of understanding research enterprise and the social world. Additionally, I was preoccupied with trying to under-stand 'how to do it', as are many novice qualitative researchers. I had a sense of something very exciting and different, but hard to 'see' and even more difficult to 'do'. To some extent I still feel this is the case, but I feel increasingly sensitised to question what other-wise may remain taken for granted and unchallenged because it appears to be so obvious.

JULIANNE   I have reached the point where I am quite comfortable with the fact that discourse analysis is not so much a technique or method for doing research, but rather an analytical approach that has impacts on every stage and step of the research process. Thus the type of questions asked, the texts generated for analysis and the way that the analysis unfolds at every point of the research process reflect discourse analysis in action. For me it is the very impossibility of achieving closure or certainty that is one of the most exciting things about discourse analysis.

CLAIRE   Another of my concerns lies in drawing on the ideas of Foucault, and identifying him as the major influence in my research approach and endeavour, and yet being relatively unfamiliar with his original texts. My anxiety was not lessened by being told that his writing was dense and 'difficult'. For the purposes of my PhD thesis, I faced this head on, acknowledged that I had not read much of Foucault's work, but drew instead from commentaries (for example Petersen and Bunton, 1997) and publications that used his ideas. In retrospect I feel that this was useful, and that

Foucault's texts themselves are indeed a difficult starting point when reading initially about discourse and positioning! However, I'm still unclear about the extent to which one should try to engage with original ideas and writing and when to do this.

JULIANNE   Of course, this is a variant of the question that is faced in any research undertaking – how much literature and theoretical underpinning is enough for any study? There is no definitive answer to this, except to say that when using discourse analysis it must be evident what theoretical influences are in play in terms of the approach to discourse analysis being undertaken. Personally, I believe that secondary sources and commentaries on major theorists are often useful places to begin, but I would also encourage the reading of the original theorists. This can be less daunting if it is undertaken with a specific purpose in mind and in conjunction with others – either fellow students or a supervisor or mentor.

CLAIRE   Having signposted our discomfort about neatly packaging this chapter and presented our arguments against doing this, perhaps we can offer a conclusion we are both happy with? Our attempt at this follows.

In summary, this chapter has illustrated the potential of discourse analysis influenced by postmodern/poststructural theoretical approaches as a means of challenging and questioning taken-for-granted aspects of health care and health care practices. There is an intimate relationship between power and knowledge constructing what is understood as natural or normal at any point in time. In the community day hospital, understandings of normal and appropriate organisation and delivery of health care were shaped by scientific/biomedical discursive frameworks. Within this organisation, whose ostensible aim was to enhance the independence and life skills of older people, an effect of this discursive frame was to constrain the ways in which older service users can be known and act. As a result, alternate subject positions and opportunities for action by older people in this setting are prohibited or simply unrecognised, because the vulnerable and 'at-risk' service user must be protected. This is to advance an alternative perspective about what otherwise might seem to be a perfectly reasonable set of assumptions about how older people should behave and be positioned in this setting. It is not to argue that necessarily one view is right and the other wrong. Rather, it is to expose that there are a number of ways of viewing the same reality, and to highlight the effect that discourses have in both constructing and maintaining that reality.

The strength of discourse analysis as presented in this chapter lies in its capacity to render problematic the assumptions, tenets and fabric of everyday life. By interrogating discursive frames that act to sustain dominant views of health and health care practices, we open up new opportunities: ones that can potentially embrace and celebrate more disparate, diverse and inclusive health-related practices for doing and being.

REFERENCES

Agger, B. (1991) 'Critical theory, poststructuralism, postmodernism: Their sociological relevance', *Annual Review of Sociology*, 17: 105–31.

Armstrong, D. (1995) 'The rise of surveillance medicine', *Sociology of Health and Illness*, 17(3): 393–404.

Armstrong, D. (1997) 'Foucault and the sociology of health and illness: A prismatic reading', in Petersen, A. and Bunton, R. (eds), *Foucault, Health and Medicine*, London: Routledge.

Ballinger, C. (1999) 'Falls and falling as explanations concerning health and self in older people', unpublished PhD thesis, Southampton: University of Southampton.

Ballinger, C. and Payne, S. (2002) 'The construction of the risk of falling among and by older people', *Ageing and Society*, 22(3): 305–24.

Cheek, J. (1997) '(Con)textualising toxic shock syndrome: Selected media representations of an emergent health phenomenon 1979–1995', *Health*, 1(2): 183–203.

Cheek, J. (2000) *Postmodern and Poststructural Approaches to Nursing Research*, London: Sage Publications.

Dew, K. (1999) 'Epidemics, panic and power: Representations of measles and measles vaccines', *Health*, 3(4): 379–98.

Fairclough, N. (1989) *Language and Power*, London: Longman.

Foucault, M. (1975) *The Birth of the Clinic*, New York: Vintage Books.

Foucault, M. (1977) *Discipline and Punish*, London: Tavistock.

Kress, G. (1985) *Linguistic Practices in Socio-cultural Practice*, Victoria: Deakin University Press.

Lupton, D. (1994) *Medicine as Culture: Illness, Disease and the Body in Western Societies*, London: Sage Publications.

Lupton, D. (1997) 'Foucault and the medicalisation critique', in Petersen, A. and Bunton, R. (eds), *Foucault, Health and Medicine*, London: Routledge.

Parker, I. (1992) *Discourse Dynamics: Critical Analysis for Social and Individual Psychology*, London: Routledge.

Parker, I. (1994) 'Discourse analysis', in Banister, P., Burman, E., Parker, I., Taylor, M. and Tindall, C. (eds), *Qualitative Methods in Psychology: A Research Guide*, Buckingham: Open University Press.

Petersen, A. and Bunton, R. (eds) (1997) *Foucault, Health and Medicine*, London: Routledge.

Petersen, A. and Lupton, D. (1996) *The New Public Health: Health and Self in the Age of Risk*, London: Sage Publications.

ACKNOWLEDGEMENTS

We would like to thank Candice Oster for her extensive and constructive comments on an earlier draft of this chapter.

15

A Case Study of Unconscious Processes in an Organisation

PAULA HYDE

Little is known about the daily work engaged in by mental health workers, yet studies of psychiatric wards have criticised them for being unkind, neglectful or cruel (see Rhodes, 1991; Walton, 2000). Other studies have suggested that mental health workers experience contradictory expectations: those of providing care for patients while containing and controlling the mentally ill on behalf of society. In spite of local and national attempts, the National Health Service (NHS), and mental health services in particular, have proved resistant to change (see Pettigrew et al., 1988).

Psychodynamic approaches to organisations allow for explanations of behaviour that may elude the participants themselves. Such approaches accept that people behave at times in ways they themselves may not understand (Gabriel and Carr, 2002). Psychodynamic research into organisations has usually taken the form of specific case studies that have sought to provide convincing reflections of social entities. The resultant theory or explanation has sometimes proved compelling, simple and useful (see Hakim, 1987; Johnson, 1975). Case studies focusing on organisations rather than individuals have been helpful in revealing social structures that would otherwise stay hidden. Examples of such case studies (Coser, 1962; Miller and Gwynne, 1972) stand out in part because their use of narrative strings together lengthy, often detailed histories.

Qualitative Research for Allied Health Professionals: Challenging Choices. Edited by Linda Finlay and Claire Ballinger.   Copyright 2006 by John Wiley & Sons Ltd.   ISBN 0-470-01963-8.

A further example of a case study that used (part of) an organisation as the unit of analysis and drew on psychodynamic methods and ideas is Isabel Menzies' classic study (Menzies, 1970). This described organisational defences used by nurses in a large London teaching hospital. In order to deflect or divert the anxiety generated by dealing with patients who were suffering and in some cases dying, nurses employed organisational defences (Menzies called these 'social defences'), which allowed them to focus on their task rather than the patients. These defences occasionally led to absurd procedures such as waking up patients to give them sleeping tablets. The simplest of decisions tended to be passed up a chain of command regardless of the skill and authority of those along the chain.

The concept of organisational defences was central to my study of the dynamics of mental health services. It seemed to offer a means of explaining behaviour that might otherwise have appeared incomprehensible. Defences against anxiety have been described in terms of individual psychology and involve the splitting of emotions to resolve internal conflict (see Klein, 1952). Among health care workers, bad feelings towards a particular patient may be projected on to outside agencies who may then be criticised. While these projections can help contain anxiety and enable staff to administer care, they may also result in states of illusory goodness and self-idealisation (Halton, 1994). Professional and hierarchical divisions within health care organisations provide fertile soil for the projection of negative feelings. As a result, professional groups and colleagues may be stereotyped and contact with them avoided to preserve self-idealisation. This interferes with collective action and cooperation between groups.

Menzies (1970) described a series of interrelated defensive routines used by nursing staff. These included splitting the nurse–patient relationship so that the nurse attended to particular tasks rather than to particular patients, thereby creating personal distance from patients. Another routine or strategy was to deny patients' individuality by treating them by category of illness. She suggested that detachment and denial of feelings were encouraged through professional training and that senior staff re-enacted repression through their disciplining and reprimanding of juniors. Ritualised activity, Menzies argued, helped to eliminate uncertainty. Nurses, too, were discouraged from using their initiative and discretion when planning work.

In their study of long-stay institutions, Miller and Gwynne (1972) described two types of defence prevalent in health care. The first was medical and aimed at prolonging life. It involved depersonalisation of the patient and increased dependence of the patient on the staff. A 'good' patient was seen as one who passively and gratefully accepted care. In contrast, the second defence was liberal. Patients were given opportunities to develop their abilities while at the same time their disabilities were denied or minimised. The 'good' patient here was seen as one who was active, happy and independent – but also doomed to fail. Roberts (1994) found that nurses were more likely to use the medical defence while other therapists were more likely to adopt the liberal one. This brought the two groups into conflict. Through a process of projection, the nurses became more rigid while the therapists grew increasingly careless of detail and inclined to be overambitious in their activity and planning. Such fragmentation along professional lines enabled staff to deflect anxiety triggered by patients.

While there is no direct parallel between individuals and institutions, psychodynamic approaches have been used to inform thinking about institutional problems (Carr and Gabriel, 2001; Hyde and Thomas, 2002, 2003). They do not claim to provide a comprehensive explanation; rather, they examine ideas that have validity at the conscious level in terms of the unconscious and hidden meaning they may carry. For example, where staff complain about computerised information systems (a conscious idea), this may imply breakdowns in interdepartmental communications (unconscious or hidden idea/meaning). Psychodynamic approaches enable these interpretations to be explored with organisational members so that their validity can be tested.

I made the decision to explore the organisational dynamics of mental health teams after conducting a similar study in a university department (Hyde, 1997). I was concerned that changes to the structure and delivery of mental health services were not leading to improvements in patient care although the circumstances of care had changed. Furthermore, I was dissatisfied with critiques that examined services from the patients' viewpoint, because they tended to portray staff simply as cruel and unkind. They did not attempt to explain why or how the staff adopted forms of behaviour that could be seen as neglectful or cruel. The pervasive nature of such experiences seemed to require explanation. I was aware, too, that I was motivated by my own belief that mental health workers (including myself) were not particularly cruel people; rather, they were people attempting to do a good job in difficult circumstances.

This chapter looks back on the study of mental health services, informed by psychodynamic theory, which I conducted between 2000 and 2002. I argue that the use of psychodynamic concepts and ideas enabled me to make interpretations that illuminated intentions and motivations otherwise hidden from the participants and from myself. Using a psychodynamic approach also enabled me to identify and elaborate on competing interpretations. I include a description of the method and theoretical approach of my study, a description of one case study from the larger study and an account of my attempts to work with competing interpretations.

METHODOLOGY: PSYCHODYNAMIC CASE STUDIES

The aim of this study was to explore how differences between mental health service contexts affected the organisational dynamics of mental health teams. This involved attempting to understand the daily work of mental health staff through observation, conversation and interviews. In order to understand what was going on I used psychodynamic concepts and techniques, in particular the concept of organisational defences, to build a picture of the daily psychological realities of work for mental health workers. Psychodynamic methods commonly involve observations and interviews and may supplement those sources with questionnaires and published data sources.

Observations involve an active process of constantly moving between detail and the general picture. Probing questions are asked of organisational members and there is a continuous attempt to classify and organise observations into basic types. Interviews then supplement this data by providing an opportunity for organisational events to be explored in depth. Such interviews are not overly structured and the interviewer is involved in active listening throughout. This enables the interviewer both to pick up new avenues for investigation and to be sensitive to their own emotional responses as well as those of the interviewee (Gabriel, 1999).

My personal experiences and emotional reactions during research encounters were used to explore and reflect on possible interpretations of what was going on. Unconscious desires and transferences mutually structure research relationships, offering the researcher the chance to explore intersubjective dynamics as well as to recognise the co-constituted nature of the research (Finlay and Gough, 2003). This process allowed for the testing of interpretations, which were developmental and responsive to discoveries made *in situ*. It was therefore important that I observed work in progress, reflected on my own emotional reactions and then used these reflections to supplement the content of conversations and interviews. I could then ask probing questions about recent events in order to explore their meaning.

During the study, psychodynamic theories were rarely made explicit unless anyone showed a particular interest. Instead, I used metaphors and comparisons to enhance interpretations as they developed. Subsequently, observations and interpretations were contrasted as part of the process of formulating and refining interpretations. In practice, some staff were more willing than others to explore their responses and any reluctance to take part was respected.

In terms of data analysis, psychodynamic approaches see analysis as an iterative process, whereby analysis may merge with data collection within interviews and conversations. Interpretations are discussed with willing organisational members, supervisors, colleagues and other experts. Where differences emerge between espoused values and daily practice, these are pointed out with a view to suggesting compromise formations. Espoused values are often printed in organisational documents or presented during formal interview, and may be contrasted with daily practice by exploring observational and conversational material.

This enquiry sought to explore mental health services without intervening purposefully to effect a change. In this respect it differed from consultancy or action research arrangements usually employed in psychodynamic studies (see Miller, 1993). The method had similarities with those arrangements, but proceeded without the imperative to effect a change. Services for people with severe and enduring mental illnesses were chosen for study because they involved staff in long-term relationships with patients and because they have been particularly criticised for poor standards of care and entrenched staff behaviour.

DOING THE RESEARCH: STUDYING MENTAL HEALTH SERVICES

The research took place within one mental health trust that covered a city and its densely populated suburbs. A case-study design was used whereby each mental health team was treated as a separate case. Following negotiations for access, each case study began with observations of daytime shifts or whole working days, depending on the opening hours of the unit. I recorded these observations in fieldwork diaries. These included records of my own emotional reactions to the environment and initial interpretations for later exploration alongside the usual records of observed events, interactions and details.

In-depth interviews were conducted with mental health service managers and commissioners and with staff, patients and carers. Opportunistic conversations were used throughout the study to explore other staff experiences linked to work processes. These conversations took place any time a participant was free and willing to talk for a short period. The information gleaned from these was compared with the findings from observations and with secondary data sources such as service information leaflets. The purpose of these comparisons was to identify differences between espoused values and daily practice that could indicate defensive processes.

The study ultimately included five case studies. At the design stage, only three studies were envisaged. However, I found it necessary to revise my categories of service settings after completing two case studies in community teams. It became clear that mental health staff were able to differentiate services into categories that were at odds with my original conception (see Figure 15.1). The two hospital settings involved in my study were the 'ward', which offered residential care, and the 'department', which offered care by appointment. Outside of the hospital, 'hostels' offered residential care and 'community mental health teams' offered care by appointment. Each case study related to

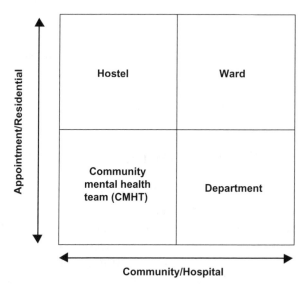

Figure 15.1 Mental health service designs

a service area that had a distinctive role in providing residential or appointment-based care and was located either within or outside the hospital environment.

My starting assumption was that different services would be linked to different organisational dynamics: for example, the ward team would establish defensive routines through daily management of the ward schedule. In contrast, I anticipated that community teams might encounter a more unpredictable daily workload, one that was less amenable to regular scheduling processes. However, given that the patient group, and to some extent the work, of each team would be similar, the organisational dynamics of different services might also exhibit common features. For example, all of them might tend to de-personalise client groups, categorising them by their condition or social circumstances.

While the theoretical grounding of the research was rarely touched on, the purpose and nature of the research were openly on view. It was possible to arrange for discussions during and following completion of the fieldwork in which participants could comment on my interpretations. Formal interviews were conducted towards the end of each case study to allow for interpretations to be explored and for work situations to be discussed. Interpretations were strengthened by contrasting interview and secondary data with observational data.

The example given below is taken from the case study that took place in a psychiatric hostel. The excerpt represents a sanitised account of what was a messy process, involving long periods of uncertainty and unexpected discoveries. These did not always originate from easily specifiable sources such as an interview quote or an observation. Rather, my past experience combined with observed events, emotional reactions and 'throwaway' comments to form ideas that could then be explored in conversation with other staff.

FINDINGS: EXCERPTS FROM THE HOSTEL CASE STUDY

The following excerpt provides a description of what happened at the hostel site. As with any summarised account, many supporting features and contextual details are missing (see Hyde, 2002, for a full account). A brief description of the case (indented account) is interspersed with my interpretations of possible organisational defences at the hostel. The description is adapted from fieldwork notes and interview transcripts.

THE HOSTEL: A REST HOME FOR THE STAFF?

The hostel offered a place of residence for up to two years for a maximum of 16 people who were experiencing long-term mental illness. All were unable to return to their former homes because of their inability to live independently, even though their condition had been stabilised on a psychiatric ward. Each resident had their own private bedroom and shared bathroom, kitchen, dining and living rooms. They were encouraged to cook their own meals and to buy their own food. The staff were keen to promote independent decision making by residents and modelled independent behaviours such as preparing breakfast or lunch, washing up and tidying dishes away. Occasionally support staff would cook breakfast for a resident as a means of enticing them out of bed before noon. Residents were encouraged to go to local day centres run by social services and to participate in community activities.

Review meetings were held for each resident every 12 weeks. The visiting consultant psychiatrist reviewed their progress and medication with staff before inviting the resident in for a discussion. As a result of the review meetings, residents were either returned to the ward or were moved on to sheltered housing.

In thinking about life at the hostel, I used the metaphor of 'rest home for the staff' to explore meanings and interpretations with staff. This metaphor sprang from my initial attempts to understand daily life in the hostel. As I saw it, the staff seemed to use the setting as if they were the residents. For example, they used the kitchen and dining room for their meals – to the exclusion of the residents. When this metaphor was presented to them, staff members offered different interpretations. One was that such 'rest home' behaviour sprang from their concern to 'model' independent behaviour for the benefit of the residents. To this end, they said, assistance was only rarely offered to residents, as it was thought to promote dependency.

Organisational defences at the hostel involved staff placing responsibility on to residents for their own behaviour while denying the residents' limitations. 'Good' residents were those who were active. By claiming to promote independence, staff could rationalise their own neglectful behaviour as constituting, or contributing to, rehabilitation. Such rationalisations are characteristic of a liberal defence (Miller and Gwynne, 1972). In the following extract, Sarah, a nurse at the hostel, shows the defence in action:

I like having the chance to sit and talk [with residents] but it's too quiet sometimes. That's the nature of rehab, you aim to enhance the quality and lifestyle. We work with the existing lifestyle, like if someone doesn't get up until 2 p.m. We don't do counselling, it's more supportive. They are enabled. They've gone through and been stabilised and sorted out where they were before. The main thing is motivating them . . . We err on the side of giving them too much [medication] to keep them stable rather than risking a relapse. Some have more side-effects. It's a balance between intrusion and caring . . .

Some long-term staff are stuck in their ways. It's a cushy place, very flexible. I mean I can commit to amateur dramatics and there aren't many places you could guarantee your shifts. With the holidays and stuff some people take the piss. They are inflexible and have a different, autocratic approach to the clients. Some came from [the old hostel] and have been here for ages. They are institutionalised staff in a hostel environment. I like the hostel work for the motivational work and the relationships.

The clash of ideals between dependence and independence was enacted in the hostel through rituals such as review meetings. Patients were sent to the hostel because they were thought to be unable to live independently in the community. Once there they were expected to be independent in caring for themselves. In spite of the emphasis placed by the staff on independent decision making by residents, the latter were excluded from the review process – where they could collaborate in deciding their treatment – until decisions about their future had already been taken. Dependent behaviour, on the other hand, was evident among long-term staff, who were said to be institutionalised.

Dependence was diverted through a process of splitting and projection. This enabled the staff to contain anxiety about their own effectiveness while working with people whose condition was likely to change only slowly. The defences also allowed staff to avoid difficult feelings associated with residents' lack of progress, as residents could be blamed for their difficulties.

Other contradictions also became apparent, as this excerpt illustrates:

The unit manager responsible for the hostel, who worked in the main hospital, suggested that the staff were highly anxious about the future of the hostel as proposals had been made to put it under independent management. In fact none of the staff demonstrated concern in this respect.

While the manager feared that the hostel would soon be put under independent management (perhaps not an accidental term), the hostel staff seemed unconcerned about their future. Practices at the hostel, such as staff adhering rigidly to their daily routines and reviews where no decisions were taken or progress registered, tended to reinforce a sense of 'stability' and changelessness. This atmosphere encouraged staff to deny the likelihood of future changes in management.

Although resources and facilities were available for the care of the residents, many of these were in fact used to benefit the staff:

> One day for me involved arriving in time for the staff handover that preceded their breakfast. All the staff ate in the shared dining room. Many residents got up later and all residents ate in the lounge. Most of the residents went out for the day after getting up and the few who remained watched television or sat in the lounge. There was a self-contained flat upstairs that had been used to enable residents to practise independent living. However, it was now used as the manager's office and staff meeting/rest rooms. Each day involved specific routines such as medication times, handovers and reviews.
>
> The staff prepared and ate meals together regularly but residents were left to their own devices. There could be a patient review or shopping outing in the afternoon but normally there was just a slow traffic of residents leaving or arriving. On this particular afternoon I sat with a resident called Florence who asked me to untangle her necklaces and then to peel a price label from the sole of her boot. After I did this, which involved me kneeling at her feet and removing the label, she spent some time talking with me about her planned move to sheltered accommodation and her feelings about leaving the hostel. Later I went into a review meeting where Andrew, one of the residents, was trying to get his medication reduced. His attempts were thwarted and he was told to take part in more community activities.
>
> I enjoyed spending time at the hostel although I felt guilty about eating food meant for the residents and for taking over their space. In this environment there was no pressure to account for myself so long as I conformed to staff routines. This felt corrupting and being there was so effortless that I feared forgetting why I was there. Often I returned home with little written down and determined to write more the next day. I spent more time at this site per week than on any of the other sites.

Florence's request that I untangle her necklaces and remove the label from the boot she was wearing involved tasks that she could easily have done independently. However, the exchange between us was meaningful in that it represented more than just the physical tasks. It established a degree of trust between us and enabled further conversations. The tasks of untangling and taking labels off may also have had symbolic meaning for Florence. She was preparing to leave the hostel and was visiting her new home, provided by a supported housing scheme, one day a week. She would be less tangled up in mental health services there and more distant from her label as a severely mentally ill person. My interaction with Florence contrasted with the reluctance of staff members, on ideological grounds, to provide assistance to the residents. Reflections on these events informed my subsequent interpretations, as did my emotional reactions to the environment.

Staff at the hostel worked over long periods with residents who were expected to progress slowly, if at all. Residents were sent to the hostel from a ward because they were judged to be unable to live independently. However, this reality was denied as staff sought to promote independent life choices, or claimed to be doing so. But when residents did attempt to take independent decisions – for example Andrew's attempt to reduce his medication – this was resisted by the staff. Hostel staff were seen by outsiders and each other as institutionalised and to some extent they behaved this way. The manager's view that the hostel would be made independent might perhaps have been an expression of her desire for the staff team to reclaim their independence. Perhaps the manager wanted them to relinquish their passive professional life, a life that could be likened to a rest or retirement home existence.

REFLECTIONS: COMPETING INTERPRETATIONS – REST HOME OR MODEL BEHAVIOUR?

In this final section, I consider how I dealt with competing interpretations that came out of the study. I also look at how interpretations of this kind might influence service design or practice development.

Psychodynamic interpretations lay at the heart of this study. I attempted to strengthen the quality of my interpretations, and maximise their coherence, by seeking clues and signs that pointed in the same direction. A better interpretation encompassed rivals by confirming, supplementing, elaborating, simplifying or superseding them. Specific outcomes were overdetermined as different indicators led to the same outcome (Gabriel, 1999, p. 272). I made a point of regularly discussing my reactions with my supervisor and with some of the people (staff and residents) at the hostel.

The metaphor of the 'hostel as rest home for staff' occurred only after I had worked with other ideas relating to how the staff dealt with boredom and their slow pace of work. I was worried about suggesting that the hostel was a rest home, because this seemed to imply that the staff were lazy. The staff responded to the metaphor in varying ways.

Some suggested that I had misinterpreted modelling behaviour, while others agreed that other staff were institutionalised. In general, however, the use of the metaphor enabled me to work across unconscious and conscious meanings without always seeking direct agreement. I was able to listen to different accounts and compare these with my observations and data from other sources.

The interpretations that arise from the psychodynamic research approach are one step removed from empirical reality and are made on the basis of numerous indicators. Many factors in evidence at the hostel pointed to the existence of a conflict between promoting independence and recognising the limitations of the residents. These instances included staff comments about not promoting dependency, my interaction with Florence, and my own sense of disquiet when participating in staff routines such as eating meals. My interpretations of these instances led me to suggest that the staff were engaged in defensive processes that enabled them to detach themselves from potential anxieties generated by their work. This detachment led the staff to treat the hostel as their own home and – to a degree – to neglect the residents.

In this setting staff went out of their way to avoid promoting dependency among residents – even though residents' lack of ability to live independently was a key criterion for their admission to the hostel in the first place. Promotion of independence was suggested by staff as the reason for their not offering help to residents. This assertion was contradicted by the failure of staff to involve residents in decision making about their care as part of their journey towards independence. Residents were excluded from the decision-making part of their review meetings, with their views being sought only at the end of such meetings. These views never seemed to be used to modify decisions that had already been made. The stated goal of promoting independence enabled the staff to distance themselves from contact with residents and could be interpreted as a rationalisation of neglect and a denial of residents' disabilities (neglect occurred where residents went short of food or where their choices were ignored). Such distancing prevented staff from experiencing anxiety about their limited ability to improve the residents' conditions, thereby shielding them from feelings of impotence.

Two competing interpretations of life at the hostel seem possible. One involves the idea of the hostel as in some ways a rest home for the staff. The other perceives the staff as model citizens, eager to demonstrate how independent living may be achieved. Which interpretation should predominate? For research within a psychodynamic perspective, importance is attached to the possibility, indeed likelihood, that there may be considerable resistance to the examination of unconscious meanings. Resistance involves refuting ideas in order that the anxiety associated with such ideas is not experienced. It also involves emotionally charged refusals to accept or hear what is being said. As such, resistance is to be distinguished from incorrect interpretations: the latter will quite properly be refuted and they normally carry less emotional energy. Resistance protects people from anxiety associated with psychological truths.

However, Gabriel (1999) warns against assuming that if research participants deny a particular interpretation, this denial is itself proof that the interpretation is correct. Instead, interpretations are corroborated by recognising the aims of resistance and the mechanisms through which it functions.

Interpretations involve heuristic methods in order to approach the psychological truths they claim to represent. For example, Florence's request for me to remove a label from her boot was interpreted by me to indicate her disentanglement from being labelled mentally ill. This involved an interpretation of an unconscious communication – one about her impending move and the jettisoning of labels. While Florence and I did not discuss any interpretations of the meaning of removing labels, we were able to explore her feelings about moving away from the hostel and her experiences of life at the hostel.

It has been my experience that interpretations are a useful way of engaging with staff about their experiences of work. Rather than being complete and self-explanatory, they offer windows of opportunity for understanding processes that are hidden and difficult to access. These processes are similar to psychotherapeutic approaches that use the examination of situations as a means of change. When accessed, defences can make understandable previously incomprehensible acts. My study enabled me to bring to the surface unconscious aspects of mental health work and to shed light on perplexing forms of staff behaviour.

My study illustrates how organisational settings can be explored to illuminate practices in terms of the meanings they incorporate. While unlikely to produce systematic solutions, such research may encourage staff to reflect on their own practice and promote service designs that allow staff to acknowledge the difficulties they face in their daily work.

REFERENCES

Carr, A. and Gabriel, Y. (2001) 'The psychodynamics of organizational change management: An overview', *Journal of Organizational Change Management*, 14(5): 415–20.

Coser, R.L. (1962) *Life on the Ward*, Michigan: Michigan State University Press.

Finlay, L. and Gough, B. (2003) *Reflexivity: A Practical Guide for Researchers in Health and Social Sciences*, Oxford: Blackwell Sciences.

Gabriel, Y. (1999) *Organizations in Depth*, London: Sage Publications.

Gabriel, Y. and Carr, A. (2002) 'Organizations, management and psychoanalysis: An overview', *Journal of Managerial Psychology*, 17(5): 348–65.

Hakim, C. (1987) *Research Design: Strategies and Choices in the Design of Social Research*, London: Routledge.

Halton, W. (1994) 'Some unconscious aspects of organizational life', in Obholzer, A. and Roberts, V.Z. (eds), *The Unconscious at Work*, London: Routledge.

Hyde, P. (1997) 'Mum, the kids and the family dog: Analysis of organisational culture', MBA dissertation, Manchester: University of Manchester.

Hyde, P. (2002) 'Organisational dynamics of mental health teams', doctoral thesis, Manchester: University of Manchester.

Hyde, P. and Thomas, A.B. (2002) 'Organisational defences revisited: Systems and contexts', *Journal of Managerial Psychology*, 17(5): 408–21.

Hyde, P. and Thomas, A.B. (2003) 'When a leader dies', *Human Relations*, 56(8): 1003–22.

Johnson, J.M. (1975) *Doing Field Research*, New York: Free Press.

Klein, M. (1952) *Developments in Psychoanalysis*, London: Hogarth Press.

Menzies, I.E.P. (1970) *The Functioning of Social Systems as a Defence against Anxiety*, London: Tavistock Institute.

Miller, E.J. (1993) *From Dependency to Autonomy*, London: Free Association Books.

Miller, E.J. and Gwynne, G.V. (1972) *A Life Apart*, London: Tavistock Institute.

Pettigrew, A.M., McKee, L. and Ferlie, E. (1988) 'Understanding changes in the NHS', *Public Administration*, 66(3): 297–317.

Rhodes, L. (1991) *Emptying Beds: The Work of an Emergency Psychiatric Unit*, Los Angeles: University of California Press.

Roberts, V.Z. (1994) 'The self-assigned impossible task', in Obholzer, A. and Roberts, V.Z. (eds), *The Unconscious at Work*, London: Routledge.

Walton, P. (2000) 'Psychiatric hospital care: A case of the more things change, the more they remain the same', *Journal of Mental Health*, 9(1): 77–88.

PART III

Presenting the Research

In this final section we consider some of the choices and dilemmas that confront you as you edge towards completing your research endeavour. In **Chapter 16**, Claire Ballinger provides enlightening ideas regarding the difficult task of demonstrating that you have carried out a rigorous research study. She also suggests some criteria by which to scrutinise and evaluate others' accounts of their research. Finally, Barbara Steward and Linda Finlay in **Chapter 17** explore some of the challenges faced by researchers who seek to disseminate their research; a stage of the research process that is all too often neglected. Specifically, they consider how to develop an argument, disseminate the research more widely and present findings effectively. The process, they say, involves both art and science; craft, inescapably, is wedded to graft.

16

Demonstrating Rigour and Quality?

CLAIRE BALLINGER

Demonstrating the rigour and quality of qualitative research poses one of the knottiest problems for us as researchers. How can we ensure that our research, in particular the analysis and interpretation it involves, has been carried out rigorously, systematically and with care? Potter and Wetherell (1987), for example, describe their approach to discourse analysis in terms of an intuitive process. However, while such claims may reflect researchers' views about the complexity of the activity, they do little to counter the criticism that qualitative research is 'merely' subjective assertion supported by unscientific method.

Many students embarking on the qualitative journey for the first time are eager to demonstrate the authority and credibility of their findings. This can stem from an anxiety about the conduct of research (often unjustified) or an awareness of being judged, for example through examination of a dissertation or thesis, or submission of a paper based on their research to a journal. Many struggle with this task and are confused and disheartened by apparently contradictory advice from textbooks. Few students, particularly at undergraduate level, represent rigour well within their work without extensive reading, support and reflection.

Qualitative researchers have a tendency to fix on concepts such as 'triangulation', 'participant validation' and 'reflexivity'. Used well these processes can help rigour and evaluation. Sometimes, however, they can

Qualitative Research for Allied Health Professionals: Challenging Choices. Edited by Linda Finlay and Claire Ballinger.   Copyright 2006 by John Wiley & Sons Ltd.   ISBN 0-470-01963-8.

be used as strategies to persuade the reader of the credibility of the work with little explanation or evidence of true engagement. The demonstration and judgement of good scholarship within qualitative research are complex issues. In this chapter, I aim to offer some guidelines about the different kinds of evaluation criteria we can bring to bear, emphasising that these depend on the epistemological position we adopt. I then offer four 'considerations' for researchers to reflect on when doing and disseminating their work. Finally, I apply these 'considerations' to two research examples.

CRITERIA FOR EVALUATION

EPISTEMOLOGICAL CHOICES INFLUENCING CRITERIA

One of the central objectives of this book is to disabuse novice researchers of the idea that 'qualitative research' represents a single set of assumptions or perspectives. As was argued in Chapter 2, researchers take different paths depending on the way they view the nature of the social world (ontology) and the way knowledge is constructed (epistemology). As the path taken influences which criteria are used to evaluate the quality of research, it is important for researchers to be clear about their position. Key distinctions centre on such questions as:

- How are reality and truth represented?
- What does the researcher claim to be accessing when generating data?
- How stable and universal do they claim their interpretation is?
- What are the roles of any fellow researchers/supervisors, particularly when interpreting data?
- How would the authors deal with competing explanations about the phenomena under investigation?
- How do their own views, agendas and experiences feature in their descriptions of their work?

(See Mason, 2002, for more examples.)

The worldview of the researcher is very rarely made explicit within their account of their work. However, hints can be found both in the style of writing and in choice of language. The following questions might provide some clues:

- Do you view the data as 'out there', waiting to be garnered or elicited? Or do you describe the bases of your interpretations as constructions, perhaps fashioned by yourself alone or jointly with research participants?

- Are you interested in participants' beliefs and attitudes? Or are you primarily concerned with their accounts and representations?
- Do additional researchers feature in the writing as providing independent evidence in support of the analysis? Or are they shown to provide guidance and help in developing analytical technique?
- Do you claim that your interpretation is the correct way of understanding the data? Or do you acknowledge that there is the potential to develop alternative explanations originating from the same data?
- Within your writing, do you stress the importance of impartiality, remaining apart from the research process and participants for fear of contaminating or biasing the process? Or do you see it as important to explain how your experiences and current roles might lead you to understand the data in particular ways?

Your answers to these questions will reveal your position on the continuum of qualitative research. For instance, are you showing yourself to be a 'realist', a 'subtle realist' or a 'relativist' (Ballinger, 2004)? Depending on your position, you will have different views as to how you can lay claim to good scholarship and rigorous research.

RELIABILITY, VALIDITY AND REALISM

The first of the three epistemological perspectives that qualitative researchers might adopt is that of the **realist**. This stance accords much more clearly with research work within a quantitative paradigm, but can also be found within qualitative work. The basic premise behind this position is that the phenomena under study exist independently of the researcher and the research endeavour. Research conducted from this position is often designed to explore very specific questions (such as comparing or contrasting, or providing evidence to explain quantitative findings). This is in contrast to research within other perspectives that generally adopt a more open or evolving design. The research question within a realist position is viewed as self-explanatory, unproblematic and perhaps emerging from a review of the literature or prior research. Within the context of the research, the question is an obvious one to pose and appeals to common sense.

In keeping with research within a quantitative paradigm, the criteria against which this form of qualitative research should be evaluated are

reliability (the degree to which findings can be deemed accurate and repeatable), **validity** (the extent to which claims for the findings truly reflect the nature of the phenomena under study) and **generalisability** (the degree to which findings have explanatory power within other contexts and situations). Reliability is often demonstrated by asking another researcher independently to code a portion of the data and comparing coding frames, while validity is sometimes established with reference to an 'expert' group. Generalisability may be enhanced by describing in detail the context and participants.

TRUSTWORTHINESS AND SUBTLE REALISM

The second position has been coined **subtle realist** by Mays and Pope (2000). An alternative description for this middle perspective is 'naturalist' (Lincoln and Guba, 1985) or 'critical realist' (Cook and Campbell, 1979). This perspective acknowledges that there is an underlying single reality that is to be explored, but argues that the various parties or players will have different views and explanations about what is happening. The job of the researcher is to explore aspects of the underlying truth through accessing these various explanations. The initial research question is therefore likely to be much more open than that found in realist research and the role of the researcher is more prominent. If we conduct research from a subtle realist position, we need to account for the ways in which we choose to access information about the phenomena, and the weight we attribute to the views of the various participants. We also need to make explicit our own agenda, preferences, choices and values and consider how these might influence our research. Hyde, in Chapter 15, carefully explains how and why she engaged in 'conversations' with research participants in order to supplement data derived from observational work. She argues that these discussions helped her not so much to validate her interpretation as to focus more sharply on defence processes in operation, and thereby develop her interpretation. She describes her research as 'co-constituted' with participants, and foregrounds her active role and strategies in the development of her interpretation.

Qualitative researchers working within a **subtle realist** position often make use of the criteria proposed by Lincoln and Guba (1985) to ensure that they carry out their research endeavour thoroughly and carefully. These criteria, developed to ensure '**trustworthiness**', comprise concepts that can be mapped against the more familiar terms ori-

Table 16.1 Positivist and naturalist criteria for determining rigour

Positivist term	Naturalistic term	Means by which rigour can be checked
Internal validity	Credibility	Prolonged involvement
		Persistent observation
		Triangulation
		Peer debriefing
		Negative case analysis
		Member checks
External validity	Transferability	Thick description
Reliability	Dependability	Enquiry audit
Objectivity	Confirmability	Audit trail

Source: Adapted from Lincoln and Guba (1985)

ginating from the quantitative paradigm. These criteria, their positivist equivalents and the means by which they can be assured are shown in Table 16.1.

Three of the most frequently mentioned strategies are **triangulation** (in which different methods are used to elicit information about the same phenomenon, and the resulting data compared to check concurrence), **thick description** (where extensive details about both the context and the participants are included) and **audit trail** (in which the researcher demonstrates how her work and thinking progressed throughout the project with the use of verifiable documents, such as a research diary, personal memos, dated computer files etc.). Stanley, for example, in her use of grounded theory in Chapter 5, describes how she produces a rich, 'thick' description via data saturation, a device particular to grounded theory in which no new codes or categories emerge from further data collection. She also writes about her use of diagrams to help her develop codes/categories, and includes her diagrams in her audit trail. This, she argues, helps to demonstrate credibility and trustworthiness (although note that this differs slightly from the formulation described earlier by Lincoln and Guba, 1985).

REFLEXIVITY, PRAGMATISM AND RELATIVISM

The third position is termed **relativist**, and is evident within the use of research methods closely associated with postmodern and poststructural ways of thinking (Cheek, 2000). Relativist qualitative researchers are likely to deny the existence of any external reality, claiming that nothing exists independently of the language and perspectives that bring phenomena into being (Edwards *et al.*, 1995). Research carried out from a relativist position is often concerned with unravelling how commonly shared worldviews are constructed and come to be accepted. Researchers of a relativist disposition will be careful not to privilege their own interpretation over competing explanations, instead presenting it as one of a number of possible representations. These researchers claim that their interpretations are personal accounts and that their own agendas, values and experiences are implicated in the production of findings. It is likely that they will **reflexively** 'write themselves into' their accounts.

Relativists may eschew any attempt to establish overarching rules, and will sometimes be suspicious of those who claim to use established criteria. However, while the logical conclusion of an extreme post-modern position might be a rejection of grand narratives or criteria, the alternative – that 'anything goes' – is also problematic. Alvesson (2002) provides a useful commentary on some of the alternative strategies proposed by postmodern researchers, including reflexivity ('conscious and systematic efforts to view the subject matter from different angles'; Alvesson, 2002, p. 171) and pragmatism (or the extent to which knowledge generated is practically useful and helpful). Later in the chapter I attempt to clarify some of the strategies fitting my relativist position that I find helpful, using my own discourse analytic work in Chapter 14 as an example.

'CONSIDERATIONS' FOR EVALUATION

The variability of perspectives in qualitative research makes it difficult to specify rules for assessing the rigour and quality of qualitative research. However, I would like to put forward what I call four 'considerations' to act as a focus for reflection. These, I argue, can be enacted in different ways, according to which of the three positions you adopt: realist, subtle realist or relativist. These are not criteria, in the usual sense of being clear standards or measures; they may more properly be viewed as pointers, as questions for you the researcher to ponder and interpret according to your own perspective.

The first consideration is **coherence**, by which I refer to the matching of such elements as research aim, view of research endeavour, researchers' accounting for their role and means by which they propose that their work should be evaluated with the particular epistemological approach adopted. Within a grounded theory account, which I suggest often, although not exclusively, lies close to the 'subtle realist' position, the aim is likely to be generating theory about concepts that are little understood or researched, with data generated by research participants as providing insights into these concepts. The researcher is likely to view their role as a collaborative one, working with participants to elicit data. However, while the data might be co-produced, they are unlikely to be described as co-constructed unless the grounded theory researcher has explicitly embraced a constructionist position (e.g. Charmaz, 2000). Evaluation criteria are likely to be similar to those suggested by Lincoln and Guba (1985), such as member checks and audit trails.

An example of a lack of coherence within a qualitative research project is where a researcher claims to be using a participatory methodology, but has the expressed aim of exploring something that derives from a health professional agenda; say, views of 'evidence-based practice'. Another anomaly within this same example might occur if the researcher is proposing that reliability is a useful concept, but asks a fellow therapist independently to code a research participant's interview transcript (rather than asking the research participant him- or herself to do so) and then compares the similarity of the coding frames.

A second consideration on which researchers might wish to reflect is **evidence of systematic and careful research conduct**. This, too, will translate differently, depending on the methodology adopted. Within our previous example of participatory research, for example, the reader should look for evidence that the researchers fully thought through the implications of how they presented themselves to potential participants, and how participants were recruited. Within a conversation analysis, the examples need to be carefully transcribed, contextualised and supported by detailed description, and the supporting text should systematically construct an explanation for the role of the particular speech device highlighted.

A third consideration that is perhaps more difficult to address is **convincing and relevant interpretation**. Within the context of discourse analysis, Potter and Wetherell (1994) describe this as 'plausibility', and using realist terminology it might be described as 'face validity'. By this I refer to recognition by the reader of the research account that the research has something significant to contribute to knowledge within the domain under investigation. As a researcher it can be difficult to ascertain if one's account is credible and compelling, particularly if the researcher has been closely involved with the research for a prolonged period. However, Potter and Wetherell (1994) suggest that presenting work to a variety of different audiences will help researchers assess how compelling their explanation is. Kvale (1996) also writes about 'communicative truth', arguing that as meaning is constructed within an interpersonal context, knowledge claims should be tested in a similar fashion. This could be through conference presentations, but also through discussion with supervisor or peers.

The final consideration is whether the **role of the researcher** is **accounted for in a way that is consistent with the orientation of the research**. Within much qualitative research this is referred to as reflection, or reflexivity, and Finlay has argued that this should be a prerequisite for all research, whether within qualitative or quantitative paradigms (Finlay, 1998).

The meaning of this strategy varies according to research tradition (see Finlay and Gough, 2003), as does the way it is enacted. Within the realist tradition, where the researcher is not considered an integral part of the research process and strives to remain objective and impartial, it would seem redundant for them to reflect on their relationship with participants, prior agendas and so on. However, considering the 'role of the researcher' within a realist writing would open up for scrutiny the ways in which the researcher endeavoured to retain objectivity and sought to maintain impartiality (for example, by using the same format of research questions within a series of semi-structured interviews).

EVALUATION IN PRACTICE

In this section I reflect on a couple of chapters from the middle section of this book to demonstrate how the above 'considerations' work in practice. The two chapters I have selected are my own postmodern/ poststructural (pm/ps) discourse analysis chapter (Chapter 14) and Linda's existential phenomenology chapter (Chapter 13), in part because we are in a position to closely interrogate our own work (and Linda has participated in this), but also because these two methodologies represent different points on the research continuum. Whereas pm/ps discourse analysis is located closer to the relativist position, existential phenomenology is epistemologically more akin to a subtle realist stance. The relevant aspects are highlighted in Table 16.2, while the text to follow explains how these address the criteria.

Table 16.2 Two worked examples illustrating considerations for determining sound scholarship

	Discourse analysis	Phenomenology
Coherence	• Aim: to look at constructions of risk in a community day hospital for older people • Research endeavour: to focus on how language and text perform particular functions • Orientation: relativist/ postmodern • Suggested criteria for evaluation: reflexivity, accounting for data in detail	• Aim: to explore the life world of a woman with MS • Research endeavour: to describe the way things appear to people • Orientation: critical (subtle) realist • Suggested criteria for evaluation: reflexivity, research participant as collaborator
Systematic and careful research conduct	• Detailed documentary evidence to support development of work • Supporting excerpts carefully contextualised, described and location within transcripts included	• 'Repeated systematic readings' of transcript • Detailed consideration of potential role of research participant
Convincing and relevant interpretation	• Interpretation worked through and supported with excerpts from data • Other studies with similar focus identified to add explanatory power and credibility	• In-depth exploration of participant's experience supported with multiple excerpts • 'Phenomenological nod'
Role of researcher	• Own agenda acknowledged through attention to reflexivity • Interpretation consistent with personal values	• 'Bracketing' of own assumptions • Nonjudgemental • Representation of interpretation as one of a number of potential explanations for data

In terms of **coherence**, I argue that both chapters stand up well. The focus on the construction of everyday life is reflected in the research aim and orientation of the pm/ps discourse analysis chapter of exploring how this is achieved through text/language, while the epistemological positioning in the phenomenological chapter is consistent with the exploration and description of the *Lebenswelt*/life world of the research participant.

The consideration of **systematic and careful research conduct** is a little more difficult to evidence. Both chapters indicate that we've taken a systematic approach. I mention inclusion of different types of data and include details of page and line in the raw data where excerpts occur. Linda talks of going through repeated analytical steps. Mention of careful note keeping, the completion of a research diary and systematic analysis is not proof in itself, and while there might be tangible evidence of these activities, the reader is unlikely to be in a position to search them out for interrogation. However, the fact that the authors mention such factors within the description of methodology is at the very least an acknowledgement that they view such activities as important and will add credibility to their accounts. It is not clear in Linda's account what tools she used.

The third consideration – **convincing and relevant interpretation** – involves perhaps even more of a personal judgement. When writing about pm/ps discourse analysis, I have worked hard to try to render my interpretation interesting and plausible. I find it challenging to present work to colleagues who are not familiar with critical theorising or postmodern thought, and sometimes struggle to make my work intelligible to a nonacademic audience. However, as an occupational therapist, I have some commitment to the practical application of my research work, and have respect for the work of Carla Willig (1999), who, almost alone among discourse analysts, has focused on the direct impact that discourse analysis research work can have on research participants. However, ultimately I believe that there are likely to be elements of my work that some readers enthusiastically embrace, and others that they discount or ignore, in part dependent on their own orientation. For her part, Linda has reflected on the lack of examples from the data within her chapter, and ponders whether this renders her interpretation less convincing. She could be criticised for focusing on literary potency rather than on systematically showing where interpretations are being made.

As a researcher of a relativist persuasion, I tend to be somewhat sceptical about phenomenological claims for data and resulting interpretation, but I find Linda's chapter (and writing generally) powerful and illuminating. I enjoy her detailed descriptions of experiences from Ann's life, interwoven with more theoretical perspectives and explanations. Perhaps the power and authority of qualitative research writing do not depend on similarity of orientation between reader and author, but rather on the way that the interpretation is warranted, and the care executed in crafting the research account.

In respect of **the role of the researcher**, I feel that Linda's chapter is particularly successful. She provides a candid account of her own struggles over how she views Ann's symptoms, and this means that she is able to 'bracket' those thoughts and perspectives deriving from her perspective as therapist. Conversely, I am not so happy with my own ability, in my chapter, to make explicit how my own agenda, experiences, even politics may be implicated in what I choose to represent as my findings, although I believe I have attended to this more successfully elsewhere (Ballinger, 2003). For me this is both an ontological and a stylistic challenge. First, while many postmodern researchers acknowledge the importance of reflexivity, one risks running counter to the postmodern project by proclaiming 'This is what I believe'. Secondly, the use of the authorial 'I' can suggest a coherence that may appear superficial and again contrary to the spirit(s!) of postmodernism! More practical constraints such as word length have forced me to be selective about what I include here.

SUMMARY

This chapter has focused on some knotty problems: how to ensure that our qualitative research is sound, how to present our work coherently and how others might be better persuaded by our account. I have emphasised how our different epistemological positions within the broad range of qualitative research approaches affect the criteria we use for evaluation. I suggested four 'considerations' for gauging the scholarship of qualitative work: coherence, systematic research conduct, convincing interpretation and account of researcher role. Reflecting on these aspects should help us conduct our work in a more rigorous fashion. It may also enhance the status and credibility of qualitative research more generally.

REFERENCES

Alvesson, M. (2002) *Postmodernism and Social Research*, Buckingham: Open University Press.

Ballinger, C. (2003) 'Navigating multiple researcher identities: Reflexivity in discourse analytic research', in Finlay, L. and Gough, B. (eds), *Reflexivity: A Practical Guide for Researchers in Health and Social Sciences*, Oxford: Blackwell Publishing.

Ballinger, C. (2004) 'Writing up rigour: Representing and evaluating good scholarship in qualitative research', *British Journal of Occupational Therapy*, 67(12): 540–6.

Charmaz, K. (2000) 'Grounded theory: Objectivist and constructionist methods', in Denzin, N. and Lincoln, Y. (eds), *Handbook of Qualitative Research*, 2nd edn, Thousand Oaks, CA: Sage Publications.

Cheek, J. (2000) *Postmodern and Poststructural Approaches to Nursing Research*, London: Sage Publications.

Cook, T. and Campbell, D.T. (1979) *Quasi-Experimentation: Design and Analysis Issues for Field Settings*, Chicago: Rand McNally.

Edwards, D., Ashmore, M. and Potter, J. (1995) 'Death and furniture: The rhetoric, politics and theology of bottom line arguments against relativism', *History of the Human Sciences*, 8: 25–49.

Finlay, L. (1998) 'Reflexivity: An essential component for all research?' *British Journal of Occupational Therapy*, 61(10): 453–6.

Finlay, L. and Gough, B. (eds) (2003) *Reflexivity: A Practical Guide for Researchers in Health and Social Sciences*, Oxford: Blackwell Publishing.

Kvale, S. (1996) *InterViews: An Introduction to Qualitative Research Interviewing*, Thousand Oaks, CA: Sage Publications.

Lincoln, Y.S. and Guba, G.G. (1985) *Naturalistic Inquiry*, Thousand Oaks, CA: Sage Publications.

Mason, J. (2002) *Qualitative Researching*, 2nd edn, London: Sage Publications.

Mays, N. and Pope, C. (2000) 'Assessing quality in qualitative research', *British Medical Journal*, 320: 50–2.

Potter, J. and Wetherell, M. (1987) *Discourse and Social Psychology: Beyond Attitudes and Behaviour*, London: Sage Publications.

Potter, J. and Wetherell, M. (1994) 'Analyzing discourse', in Bryman, A. and Burgess, R.G. (eds), *Analyzing Qualitative Data*, London: Routledge.

Willig, C. (1999) *Applied Discourse Analysis*, Buckingham: Open University Press.

17

Disseminating the Research: Towards Knowledge

LINDA FINLAY AND BARBARA STEWARD

Having completed your research – perhaps collecting a degree as a result – what do you do now? Sadly, all too many dissertations languish on university library bookshelves figuratively gathering dust. Their authors, most likely exhausted after making such a big commitment and with new priorities, somehow turn their backs on their own research. Perhaps they are uncertain of what steps to take to present their research to an audience beyond their research supervisor, examiners and the odd interested colleague.

While such responses are completely understandable, what a waste of all those discoveries, that new and exciting knowledge! The recent 'Standards of Proficiency' (Health Professions Council, 2004) emphasise that therapists have an obligation not only to engage in research but also to share their findings towards informing and improving practice in a wider context. It surely behoves us to disseminate the results of our research as widely as possible. After all, engaging in research is geared to more than simply jumping through academic hoops or advancing academic careers. Research is there for us to use or apply in some way. In the case of research carried out by health professionals, the findings can enhance practice, provide evidence of effectiveness or inform professional education. But this is only possible if the research is successfully disseminated. Doing this, however, is easier said than done.

Qualitative Research for Allied Health Professionals: Challenging Choices. Edited by Linda Finlay and Claire Ballinger.   Copyright 2006 by John Wiley & Sons Ltd.   ISBN 0-470-01963-8.

This chapter explores issues around disseminating research by looking at three particular challenges:

- developing an argument that convinces a wider audience of the value and interest of your research;
- disseminating research more widely;
- presenting findings effectively in papers and presentations.

THE CHALLENGE OF DEVELOPING A CONVINCING ARGUMENT

As the contributors to this book have shown, qualitative research presents a range of complex problems and choices. These have to be fully addressed and worked through in order to convey the nature, rigour and implications of the evidence used. Unlike quantitative approaches where statistical analysis forms the core of the results, qualitative approaches are more difficult to account for and justify. As qualitative researchers, we have to explain our position within the study and justify our subjectivity. We must find an appropriate way to record and explain complex, messy findings. We must also analyse the claims we are making and question what they are based on. Perhaps most important of all, we have to provide evidence of the trustworthiness of our research and argue a case for its value.

Barbara, one of the authors of this chapter, reflects below on the challenges:

> Good research makes statements that go beyond simple answers to research questions. It makes claims about how we have created new knowledge or confirmed or challenged existing knowledge.
>
> Like many researchers, when I came to the end of my research I found that I was reticent about making claims for my research. I was overcome by a mixture of modesty and fear of sticking my neck out. I was highly conscious of how so much effort had resulted in such an apparently small – insignificant? – nugget of knowledge. I was also surprised that so little help was on offer in the literature about making the step between doing the analysis and presenting the research towards making knowledge. Punch states: 'researchers should articulate their conclusions, and describe their meaning in the worlds of ideas and the actions they affect' (Punch, 1998, p. 277). But there was little guidance on how this might be achieved.
>
> Now, having gained some experience, the guidance I would offer is to answer what I call the 'so what?' questions: So what does it all seem to mean? So what ways can I devise to frame my evidence of, and in, the world of my study? So what do I understand now and what has changed

from what I thought before? So what difference has the research made to my beliefs and practice or those of other people involved?

Mason (2002) provides some wise advice on arguing the case for your research. She suggests that because the arguments developed in the discussion are relational, planning how to put them across in written or verbal presentations requires special attention. As she notes, this raises 'practical as well as epistemological questions about how to get qualitative data into an argument, how to select, represent and "display" them, and so on, in ways that will be coherent, meaningful and ultimately convincing' (Mason, 2002, p. 183).

These are difficult issues, demanding that careful thought be given to how research is explained and justified and how its usefulness and trustworthiness can be demonstrated. The audience needs to be provided with sufficient detail to enable them to be convinced of its quality. Knowing your audience is vital to making your case and presenting it in an accessible way. It is important, too, that your presentation takes into account your audience's prior knowledge of the topic and familiarity with the research methodology.

A strong, persuasive argument is central to the effective presentation of research. Mason (2002, pp. 176–7) describes four ways of arguing, each of which reaches back to or connects with the epistemological claims of your research:

- **Arguing evidentially** ('I can make this argument because I can show you the relevant evidence') . . .
- **Arguing interpretively or narratively** ('I can make this argument because I can show you that my interpretation or my narrative is meaningful or reasonable') . . .
- **Arguing evocatively or illustratively** ('I can make this argument because I can evoke understanding or empathy in you, or because I can provide meaningful illustration') . . .
- **Arguing reflexively or multivocally** ('I can make this argument because I can make you aware of a meaningful range of perspectives, experiences and standpoints, including my own')

When arguing evidentially, we need to demonstrate that we've marshalled our evidence systematically. We need, too, to be clear about how our data constitutes evidence. Chapters 5, 6, 7 and 8 in Part II of this book have argued in this way, using quotes and illustrative examples. If we are arguing interpretively or narratively, we seek to show that our interpretations are both reasonable and suitably nuanced. Chapters 10, 11 and 15 illustrate this approach in action. Arguing evocatively or illustratively involves getting readers/the audience to understand experientially – to 'feel' the power of our research, as Chapter 13 has sought to illustrate. When arguing reflexively or multivocally, our aim is to show sensitivity to the co-constructed nature of our research and our willingness to critique our positions. While all the chapter authors in this book have been reflexive, Chapters 9, 12 and 14 are particularly good illustrations of this approach.

These differences in approach imply different understandings of what constitutes data, 'truth' and theory building. Such differences go to the heart of what we're trying to do in our 'research-as-science'. Is our purpose to follow the model of natural science or do we wish to endorse what we might describe as moral science (that is, science concerned with human potential) or even political science, seeing our work as part of a process of social change (Wetherell, 1996)?

Mason (2002) goes on to suggest a number of steps towards making a good argument. Her recommendations can be summarised thus:

- Select the data to include in your argument carefully. Are you seeking to use data in a realist or interpretivist way? Is it illustrative or constitutive of your argument?
- Use that data imaginatively. As Mason (2002, p. 185) observes, 'researchers who wish to argue evocatively, either because they want to argue about the senses or things that do not exist in words . . . or because in a postmodern vein of multivocality they take issue with the idea that a researcher has authority to speak for others . . . , will certainly be interested in a range of forms of expression.'
- Check that you are convinced by your argument by putting your assumptions and analysis to the test. Make sure they've been transparently and systematically constructed.

Having developed a convincing argument about the research and worked out what our research contributes to the wider world, we next face the challenge of how to share our message.

THE CHALLENGE OF DISSEMINATING RESEARCH MORE WIDELY

Richardson throws down the gauntlet when she asserts:

> Qualitative work could be reaching wide and diverse audiences, not just devotees of the topic or the author. It seems foolish at best, and narcis-

sistic and wholly self-absorbed at worst, to spend months or years doing research that ends up not being read and not making a difference to anything but the author's career. (Richardson, 1994, p. 517)

Working out how to disseminate our research turns on two basic questions: who we are and where we seek to have impact. If you are a clinician doing applied research, you'll especially want to communicate with colleagues, managers and/or service users. Peer presentations, conferences, research forums and local interest groups will probably be your first port of call. If you're in the academic world, you'll have an eye to research assessment exercises (RAEs) and will be working to publish articles in prestigious journals. The directive 'publish or perish' is a spectre that looms large for academics in the increasingly competitive university world. While we know that we 'should' publish our research, it is quite another matter to actually get the stuff accepted for publication. (It is beyond the scope of this chapter to address this, but there are helpful books on writing up and getting published: for instance Wolcott, 1990 and Richardson, 1994).

Watching experienced presenters at conferences can be an instructive and useful first step. As you observe them in action, ask yourself questions. What is it that they're doing that makes their presentation effective and catches interest? Equally, what are poor or less effective presenters doing that should be avoided? Collaborating with supervisors and other more experienced colleagues in writing or making presentations can help, too. Good experience can also be gained from peer presentations. These can help to nurture confidence and develop critical debating skills. Similarly, much can be learnt from acting as a peer reviewer appraising proposed journal articles.

The 'W' questions (to whom? what? where? why?) can serve as useful prompts as you think about how to disseminate your research more widely. For example, Walker (2005) highlights the 'where?' question when discussing the choice before researchers of publishing only in the *British Journal of Occupational Therapy* or of publishing more widely.

Below, the authors of this chapter each reflect on the choices they've made on the basis of their individual priorities:

BARBARA   When I was a clinician I was concerned to share my research through publications and conference presentations, but uncertain about which to submit to and easily discouraged by reviewers' comments. I experienced strong feelings of vulnerability when these papers were published when I had to defend my ideas following a presentation. Collaborating with more experienced presenters and attending conferences within other disciplines enabled me to develop my own style. I found myself better able to plan which elements of my work to present to a particular audience. I began to realise that my 'small nugget' of information was interesting and challenging to others. In my role as research therapist I have been able to share these experiences with new authors and presenters. I have encouraged them to see the review process (including critical comments from colleagues) in a positive light. Having been in a position to disseminate my research to government, business and academic audiences, I've found that the feedback I've received from each has provided me with new insights. The challenge is always to make my theories on health and occupation accessible and relevant.

LINDA   My main challenge is strategic in nature: it involves working out what to publish and where. Should I publish in practice-oriented journals or more research-oriented ones? Should I stick with journals geared to UK practice or take the more difficult path of trying to get published in international journals? A particular challenge remains that of how to recycle and repackage my research for different journals. There seems to be an ever-expanding pool of messages to pull out. Regarding my work on reflexivity, for instance, my first article (in which I introduced the concept) appeared in the *British Journal of Occupational Therapy*. I subsequently elaborated by unpacking different variants of reflexivity in journals such as *Qualitative Research*, publications that have a wider audience. I'm continuing to develop this work and am now concentrating on phenomenological variations for scholarly phenomenological journals. In all these different articles I've drawn on similar ideas, data and examples. The hard part is to find the style and storyline appropriate for a particular audience – and to ensure that the story is always told in meaningful and interesting ways.

THE CHALLENGE OF PRESENTING FINDINGS EFFECTIVELY

Perhaps the biggest challenge we face when disseminating our research is overcoming constraints of time and space. As journal articles are usually limited to between 6000 and 7000 words, it is indeed a challenge to boil down an 80,000-word dissertation to these dimensions. For conference presentations, meanwhile, we may find ourselves allocated just 10 or 15 minutes in which to present our research. Though people try valiantly, it is not possible to squeeze a detailed look at methodology, method and findings together with a discussion into such a thin time slot. What is always required is a radical repackaging of our research to suit the forum. In short, we need to learn how to 'dedissertationalise' our work (Wolcott, 1990)!

Repackaging your research material entails thinking about how to present it. Presenting at conferences is one clear-cut choice, while setting out to write a journal article is another. Box 17.1 offers six key tips for presenting findings effectively, whether this entails writing a journal article or presenting a conference paper.

Whatever forum you choose to present in, and however you do it, allow yourself plenty of time to prepare for the presentation. It is amazing to see how your own knowledge and understanding evolve as you work on presenting your research. Your message needs time to co-alesce. It is helpful here to rehearse your presentation. If you're going to give a talk, then practise it with an eye to your time constraints. Think about how to pace it, making sure you build in time for questions or interruptions if appropriate. If you're writing a piece, be prepared to work through numerous successive drafts as you hone your ideas and your writing. When Linda writes a journal article, for example, she redrafts it several times, often changing her structure and content

---

Box 17.1   Six tips for presenting research

1. Find a specific focus   You want to find a 'storyline' that will hook the reader/listener in. Does your research address a particular problem? Is there a particular line of argument you're trying to put forward? Are you linking into a topical debate? Are you challenging some existing practice? It can help to begin with one or two sentences that will capture personal interest. For example, you might link your research with something topical from the media or ask your audience a question that your talk might then go on to address.

2. Be selective   Home in on aspects of your research that might be particularly relevant and significant. It can be useful, for instance, to limit yourself to just three key points. (This tip is also useful to remember if you're using slides or making OHP

acetates – don't indulge in information overload.) While you want some quotes and illustrations, use these judiciously. You won't be able to present the entirety of your research, so what message do you want to highlight?

3. Keep your audience in sight   Whom are you writing for or speaking to? What might they be interested in learning? If your audience is made up of other practitioners or policy makers, then you need to relate your findings to practice or policy issues. A more academic audience will expect more theory or an interesting slant on methodology. It's important not to make a lay audience feel threatened or alienated by your research.

4. Write/speak in an interesting way   There are, of course, no hard-and-fast rules about what makes an interesting presentation. To some extent 'interesting' is in the eye (or ear) of the beholder. However, you can aim to make some impact. The best presentations seem to highlight findings that are unexpected, humorous, poignant or particularly intriguing. Silverman (2000, p. 270) advises budding authors to 'tease, entice and puzzle'.

5. Adopt an appropriate style and tone   A scholarly journal article demands a style that would be inappropriate for an opinion piece, though both may be based on the same evidence. Stylistic decisions rest on what you want to say, to whom, in what context and within what sort of relationship. Ask yourself if you are principally out to inform, debate, impress or instruct. It can help dramatically if a supportive colleague or friend gives you critically supportive feedback. You should read the journals you intend to submit to in order to know where your work will best fit. See their author guidelines as an aid to publication rather than a straitjacket.

6. Be creative   Might there be more creative, fresher ways of presenting your research? Look on your research as 'wet clay' (Richardson, 1994, p. 523), there to be shaped! Poetry, drama, film, fiction and other polyvocal experimental forms, judiciously used, may prove more powerful than traditional presentation modes. By problematising notions of 'truth' and 'validity' (Richardson, 1994), such forms nudge us towards recognition of the constructed nature of all texts.

radically in response to feedback from others. She also expects to do further redrafting after it has been peer reviewed; articles are rarely accepted by journal editors straight off.

This chapter has explored some of the challenges faced by researchers when seeking to disseminate their research. Presenting your research – and doing it well – takes time. It involves art and science; craft and graft. The reward comes from knowing you have contributed something of value; that you have taken part in 'making knowledge'. When your findings are applied in some way to practice, or others are appreciative of the insights your work offers, you know your research journey has been worthwhile.

Richardson (1994) suggests that learning to write (and we'd add learning to present research) can be seen as part of a process of enquiry. She argues that researchers' self-knowledge and understanding of their topic develop through writing. She seeks to 'encourage individuals to accept and nurture their own voices' (Richardson, 1994, p. 523).

Ultimately, presenting and disseminating your research is a new journey in itself – a process of discovery, of ourselves and of knowledge. As you take up opportunities to share your research more widely, we hope that you, too, will value and nurture your own individual voice.

REFERENCES

Health Professions Council (2004) 'Standards of proficiency', accessed at www.hpc-uk.org/publications/standards.htm, 20 March 2005.

Mason, J. (2002) *Qualitative Researching*, 2nd edn, London, Sage Publications.

Punch, K. (1998) *Introduction to Social Research: Quantitative and Qualitative Approaches*, London: Sage Publications.

Richardson, L. (1994) 'Writing: A method of inquiry', in Denzin, N.K. and Lincoln, Y.S. (eds), *Handbook of Qualitative Research*, Thousand Oaks, CA: Sage Publications.

Silverman, D. (2000) *Doing Qualitative Research: A Practical Handbook*, London: Sage Publications.

Walker, M. (2005) 'Time to make an impact', *British Journal of Occupational Therapy*, 68(2): 55.

Wetherell, M. (1996) 'Defining social psychology', in Sapsford, R. (ed.), *Issues for Social Psychology*, Milton Keynes: Open University.

Wolcott, H. (1990) *Writing up Qualitative Research*, Newbury Park, CA: Sage Publications.

Glossary

Please note that the concepts, approaches and methodologies identified below are not the only frameworks within which qualitative enquiry can be carried out. We have selected these on the basis that they are the ones most commonly used within qualitative allied health research.

Action research Action research addresses the specific aim of improving the quality or performance of an organisation or service as an intrinsic part of the research process. This process typically involves generating data about existing performance, identifying and implementing agents for change, and evaluating outcomes. A range of both quantitative and qualitative methods may be employed to this end.

Biographical-narrative-interpretive research (BNIR) BNIR is a highly structured research approach, drawing on hermeneutic phenomenological traditions, in which the research participants' constructed meanings are investigated through the generation of narratives. These narratives are typically elicited through a series of interviews in which process and themes are progressively clarified. Analysis may involve joint interpretation through use of research panels.

Biographical research Biographical research is concerned with the individual life experiences of research participants. Such approaches may involve asking participants to write their life stories, or to share these stories over the course of one or more interviews. Biographical researchers orientate to the words used by participants (for example in presenting findings) and the individual meanings attributed to them. Attention is paid to the chronology of life events and how these are culturally and socially influenced.

Qualitative Research for Allied Health Professionals: Challenging Choices. Edited by Linda Finlay and Claire Ballinger. Copyright 2006 by John Wiley & Sons Ltd. ISBN 0-470-01963-8.

Case study   Case study research involves the exploration of a small number of cases (which may be individual participants, events or organisations), selected on the basis of offering rich or pertinent findings in order to address the research question. Multiple methods may be used to generate data (for example observation and interview) and the report of the research will include detailed contextual description.

Constructivism   Constructivism is a paradigm most commonly used in ethnographic, phenomenological and narrative research. This research position rejects the idea that we can verify knowledge by reference to the 'real' outside world (i.e. we do not discover an objective ontological reality). Knowledge is not passively received either through the senses or by way of communication, but is actively built up by a perceiving, cognitive 'subject'.

Conversation analysis   Conversation analysis employs observational methods in a highly systematic way in order to obtain detailed descriptions of social interaction. The foci of conversation analysis can include ordinary conversation, institutional interactions and interactions between individuals and technology, and also addresses nonverbal communications. Transcription tends to be extremely detailed, including such features as volume, pauses and inflexion.

Cooperative enquiry   An approach whereby people who share similar research interests and concerns work collaboratively together, to create joint research agendas, ways of exploring, processes of reaching understanding and capturing outcomes of research. This approach in particular challenges the traditional roles in the research process of 'researcher' and 'research participant'. Instead, the two roles are often combined with the participant becoming a 'co-researcher'. See **Participatory research**.

Critical approaches   Critical researchers challenge the 'taken for granted' within social contexts. They are concerned with unpacking how concepts come to be constructed as common sense, and exploring the social implications of such common and unproblematic views. Researchers employing critical approaches also seek to explore the perspectives of those who are disenfranchised by these widely shared understandings.

Critical realism   A philosophical position that acknowledges there is a pre-existing external reality and that it is the purpose of social enquiry to explore this. It also recognises that this reality is mediated through and by individual experience and representation, and is socially situated. Meanings are understood to be somewhat fluid. See **Subtle realism**.

Discourse analysis   Discourse analytic research approaches share a focus on talk and texts as constructing social truths, and also being indicative of wider systems of meaning that inform how the social world is understood. There are many different types of discourse analysis, perhaps the two most widely used in health research being postmodern/poststructural (influenced by Foucauldian ideas of power/knowledge) and the more linguistically oriented form, which draws on conversation analysis and ethnomethodology.

Epistemology   Epistemology is a philosophical concept that is concerned with the constitution of knowledge: what it is like, from where it is derived and how it may be explored. It poses such questions as: What understanding is the researcher aiming for? What kind of knowledge can be gained?

Ethnography   A research approach originally deriving from social anthropology, ethnography is a description and interpretation of a cultural group or social system. It aims to describe a group or culture through fieldwork involving prolonged immersion in the context of interest, typically through participant observation. The researcher investigates typical behaviours, customs, meanings, interactions and day-to-day lives in general.

Ethnomethodology   Ethnomethology is the study of everyday practices and understandings through which people make sense of others' actions, and which shape their own. The aim is to describe how taken-for-granted 'rules' lie behind everyday conversations and interactions.

Existentialism   Existentialism is a philosophical theory that emphasises the existence of individuals as active, free agents responsible for what they make of themselves. Kierkegaard, Nietzsche, Heidegger and Sartre were the major thinkers connected with this movement. Heidegger and Sartre developed their own phenomenological existential analyses concerned with *Being*, authenticity and freedom.

Feminist research   This approach is used to describe research that specifically addresses the position of women in social contexts, with recognition of the inherent sexism in many organisations and institutions. The purpose of feminist research is to establish non-exploitive, collaborative relationships that aim to 'give voice to' marginalised groups. Feminist researchers aim to conduct potentially transformative research. See **Critical approaches**.

Grounded theory   This term describes research approaches in which theory is inductively built from, and grounded in, data. The researcher aims to generate a theory or analytical schema that explains some process or aspect of the social world. A 'constant comparative method' ensures that data generation and analysis occur concurrently, and that analytic concepts are systematically honed, becoming progressively more abstract. Glaser and Strauss, the originators of this methodology, diverged in their development of grounded theory in later years. Glaser's approach to grounded theory emphasises rigorous and systematic conduct of research and analysis, while Straussian grounded theory draws heavily on interpretive influences.

Hermeneutics   Hermeneutics is concerned with the theory and practice of interpretation. It emerges out of the work of philosophers such as Gadamer, Dilthey, Ricoeur and Heidegger. Gadamer, for instance, argues that in interpreting a text, we cannot separate ourselves from the meaning we gain; understanding always involves interpretation.

Interpretative phenomenological analysis (IPA)   This variant of phenomenology aims to explore individuals' perceptions and experiences. Taking an idiographic approach, the focus is on individuals' cognitive, linguistic, affective and physical being. IPA involves a two-stage interpretation process as the researcher tries to make sense of participants' sense making. See **Phenomenology**.

Interpretivism   A research position that posits that objective understanding is impossible, as perceptions and experiences mediate how phenomena are both represented (for example by research participants) and comprehended (for example by researchers). What is true for me may not be true for you – it all depends on our perspective. The interpretivist researcher recognises that they are a part of the world they are studying.

Method   Research methods are the procedures and means of collecting or generating data within a research study. In isolation, research methods are often relatively atheoretical, being focused on the practicalities of obtaining raw information for analysis.

Methodology   The general approach to the research endeavour, underpinned by theoretical and philosophical ideas, determining the focus of the study, methods to be employed, form of analysis and how the researcher views their own position and role.

Narrative research   This approach to research holds that the narrative, or storyline, in a research participant's account is organised in particular ways that facilitate understanding or meaning ascribed by the author (i.e. the participant). Narrative researchers treat narratives as the organising basis of human action. Through our stories (which reflect culturally available narratives) we make sense of our experience.

Naturalism   Naturalism is the philosophical view that research should remain true to the nature of the phenomenon under study. It proposes that, as far as possible, the social world should be studied in its 'natural' state. Representing a range of research methodologies such as ethnography and ethnomethodology, it aims to describe and interpret the social world posing research questions that ask 'how?' and 'what?'.

Ontology   A philosophical idea concerned with the nature of the social world: what it comprises, the objects within it and the relationships between those objects. Is something 'real' or is it in the mind of the actors? Ontology means questioning the nature of ourselves as social beings and questioning what it means to be.

Paradigm   A paradigm is a philosophy or 'worldview'. See **constructivism**, **critical approaches**, **positivism**, **postpositivism** and **poststructuralism** for examples of research paradigms.

Participant validation   Participant validation is advocated within some research paradigms as a way of testing the validity, or truth, of one's research findings. According to this technique, emergent findings are returned to those who participated in the research study to ensure that these findings reflect the meanings intended by participants.

Participatory research   Participatory research places a strong emphasis on participation and empowering potentially disadvantaged groups. It involves a research approach that aims to demystify the research process, therefore enabling nonresearchers to engage in, use and benefit from research endeavour. Often, research participants are invited to become 'co-researchers'. See **Cooperative enquiry**.

Personal construct research   Personal construct research is a research approach used in psychology that is based on George Kelly's personal construct theory. A person's constructs are elicited through using the 'repertory grid technique'. Analysing these, the researcher aims to understand the way research participants construe (i.e. think and feel about) their world.

Phenomenology   Phenomenology is an umbrella term encompassing both a philosophical movement and a range of research approaches. In general, phenomenology is the study of phenomena: their nature and meanings. The focus is on the way things appear to us through experience or in our consciousness. The phenomenological researcher aims to provide a rich textured description of 'lived experience'. See **Existentialism.**

Positivism   Positivism is a perspective that views testing, observation and measurement as central to the establishment of scientific knowledge. Positivists hold that concepts that can't be proved empirically are not deemed worthy of scientific study. See **Realism.**

Postmodernism   Postmodernism is a loose collective of positions and approaches that challenge the stability and grand theory of modernity, favouring instead ambiguity, multiplicity and focused detail in preference to meta-narratives. See **Poststructuralism.**

Postpositivism   Postpositivism is a philosophical position that holds that the central mission of scientific endeavour is to describe and document reality, while acknowledging the fallibility of measurement and the role of theory within scientific knowledge. Postpositivist researchers recognise the challenge of studying a complex social world that cannot be reduced to simple objective measures.

Poststructuralism   Poststructuralism is a collective term for a group of perspectives that provide a critique of the advancement and permanency of scientific knowledge, instead valuing diversity, difference and multiplicity, with a particular focus on texts and representation. See **Postmodernism.**

Psychodynamic research approaches   These research approaches are based on the work of Freud and other psychodynamic theorists that aim to explore unconscious developmental processes through processes of observation, interview or analysis of written accounts. Psychodynamic concepts and approaches can be applied at the level of the individual, group or institution.

Realism   Realism is a philosophical perspective that holds that it is possible to acquire objective knowledge, through research, about a permanent and stable reality. The world, according to realists, is made up of structures and objects that have cause–effect relationships with each other. The aim of realist research is to study the 'real' world 'out there'.

Reflection   Reflection can be defined as 'thinking about' something after the event. Researchers commonly reflect on their research through the use of reflective diaries that record their thoughts, feelings and general observations during and after fieldwork.

Reflexivity   Reflexivity is self-aware, critical reflection of the ways in which the researcher might have influenced the objectives, process and outcomes of the research. In contrast to reflection, reflexivity involves a more immediate, dynamic and continuing self-reflection. Versions of reflexivity are practised that range from using it as a methodological tool (to audit the research and ensure its 'truth') to exploiting it as a way of undermining truth claims.

Relativism   Relativism is a philosophical position that holds that all perspectives are of equal value and that it is impossible to distinguish good and bad, right and wrong. An extreme relativist would propose that there is no distinction between what is real and what is not, as 'reality' can only be apprehended through, and is therefore mediated by, personal perception and/or language use.

Social constructionism   Social constructionism is a philosophical, social psychological perspective that focuses on the ways in which social phenomena are collectively represented (for example through visual characterisation or texts) and the ideological interests motivating these representations. This perspective argues that conventional views of a person as having a core personality are misleading. Instead, identities are seen to emerge through discourse and relationships within a social context.

Subtle realism   Subtle realism is a research position that assumes that, while there is an underlying social reality, different researcher and participant perspectives allow different and partial views of that reality. Meanings are understood to be somewhat fluid. See **Critical realism**.

Symbolic interactionism   Symbolic interactionism is a social psychological theoretical perspective originally connected with the work of George Herbert Mead and the Chicago School. Symbolic interactionists understand social reality as a complex network of interactions between interpreting people. From this perspective, people's self-definitions are shaped by others. We are seen to act on the basis of how we perceive that others think and feel about us.

Triangulation   Triangulation of research methods is a technique advocated within more realist research traditions that aims to test the validity of research findings. This is done by comparing the outcomes of using different methods of exploring the same phenomenon to check that they are all consistent.

Trustworthiness   Trustworthiness is a means of viewing and checking issues around quality and rigour within qualitative research. Qualitative researchers often reject criteria of validity, reliability and generalisability traditionally used for quantitative research. Instead, a range of different criteria are put forward, including trustworthiness, credibility, plausibility and communicative validity.

Index
